High-Yield Heart

Y0-CAS-344

High-Yield Systems
High-Yield Heart

Ronald W. Dudek, PhD
Brody School of Medicine
East Carolina University
Department of Anatomy and Cell Biology
Greenville, North Carolina
dudekr@mail.ecu.edu

◆ LIPPINCOTT WILLIAMS & WILKINS
A **Wolters Kluwer** Company

Philadelphia • Baltimore • New York • London
Buenos Aires • Hong Kong • Sydney • Tokyo

Acquisitions Editor: Betty Sun
Managing Editor: Elena Coler
Marketing Manager: Emilie Linkins
Production Editor: Julie Montalbano
Designer: Doug Smock
Compositor: Circle Graphics, Inc.
Printer: Courier—Kendallville

Copyright © 2006 Lippincott Williams & Wilkins

351 West Camden Street
Baltimore, MD 21201

530 Walnut Street
Philadelphia, PA 19106

All rights reserved. This book is protected by copyright. No part of this book may be reproduced in any form or by any means, including photocopying, or utilized by any information storage and retrieval system without written permission from the copyright owner.

The publisher is not responsible (as a matter of product liability, negligence, or otherwise) for any injury resulting from any material contained herein. This publication contains information relating to general principles of medical care that should not be construed as specific instructions for individual patients. Manufacturers' product information and package inserts should be reviewed for current information, including contraindications, dosages, and precautions.

Printed in the United States of America

Library of Congress Cataloging-in-Publication Data

Dudek, Ronald W., 1950-
  High-yield heart / Ronald W. Dudek.
    p. ; cm. — (High-yield systems)
  ISBN 0-7817-5568-9
  1. Cardiology—Examinations, questions, etc. I. Title. II. Series.
  [DNLM: 1. Heart—Examination Questions. 2. Heart Diseases—Examination Questions. WG 18.2 D844h 2006]
  RC669.2 .D83
  616.1′2′0076—dc22
                                                          2005023080

The publishers have made every effort to trace the copyright holders for borrowed material. If they have inadvertently overlooked any, they will be pleased to make the necessary arrangements at the first opportunity.

To purchase additional copies of this book, call our customer service department at **(800) 638-3030** or fax orders to **(301) 824-7390**. International customers should call **(301) 714-2324**.

Visit Lippincott Williams & Wilkins on the Internet: http://www.LWW.com. Lippincott Williams & Wilkins customer service representatives are available from 8:30 am to 6:00 pm, EST.

05 06 07 08 09
1 2 3 4 5 6 7 8 9 10

Preface

A Focused Curriculum is a curriculum whereby students are immersed in one basic science discipline (e.g., Histology) for a concentrated period of time when Histology is covered from A to Z. A Systems-based Curriculum is a curriculum whereby students are immersed in one system (e.g., Cardiology system) for a concentrated period of time when all basic science disciplines of the Cardiology system are covered (e.g., Embryology, Histology, Physiology, Pharmacology).

The High-Yield Systems series addresses a problem endemic to U.S. medical schools and medical students using a Focused Curriculum. After completing a Focused Curriculum, the medical student is faced with the daunting task of integrating and collating all the basic science knowledge accrued from the Focused Curriculum into the various systems. For example, a medical student wanting to review everything about the heart will find the information scattered in his or her Embryology notes, Histology notes, Physiology notes, Pharmacology notes, and so on. The High-Yield Systems series eliminates this daunting task for the medical student by bringing together the Embryology, Gross Anatomy, Radiology, Histology, Physiology, Pathology, Microbiology, and Pharmacology of the heart all in one clear concise book.

The High-Yield Systems series has uses for the following student groups:

1. First-year medical students in a Focused Curriculum who want to get a head start on the inevitable integration and collation process of all the information learned in a Focused Curriculum into systems
2. First-year medical students in a Systems-based Curriculum, who will find this series a natural textbook for a Systems-based Curriculum
3. Medical students preparing for Step 1 of the USMLE where the questions are becoming increasing more systems-based than discipline-based
4. Second-year medical students for whom the curriculum is much more systems-based as Pathology covers the pathology of each system as a block (e.g., pathology of the lung, pathology of the heart, pathology of the kidney, etc.)
5. Senior medical students who may want to quickly review all aspects of lung function before starting a rotation in Cardiology, for example
6. Recent medical graduates who may want to quickly review all aspects of lung function before starting a residency in a specialization such as Cardiology

In the High-Yield Systems series, the student will find the same painstaking attention given to include high-yield information as that found in other High-Yield books. However, the breadth of information has been expanded somewhat to cover some baseline information without which a complete understanding of the system would be difficult.

The High-Yield books based on the presentation of high-yield information that is likely to be asked on the USMLE has clearly been an asset to the medical student. However, after writing many High-Yield books, I have found that high-yield information can also be presented in a highly efficient manner. In the High-Yield Systems series, the student now gets the benefit of both high yield and high efficiency in their studies.

I appreciate any feedback and can be contacted at dudekr@mail.ecu.edu.

Table of Contents

Chapter 1

Embryology

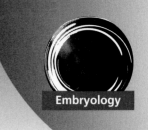

I Formation of the Heart Tube *(Figure 1-1A–D)*

Lateral plate mesoderm (at the cephalic area of the embryo) splits into a somatic layer and a splanchnic layer, thus forming the **pericardial cavity.** Precardiac mesoderm is preferentially distributed to the splanchnic layer and is now called **heart-forming regions (HFRs).** As lateral folding of the embryo occurs, the HFRs fuse in the midline to form a continuous sheet of mesoderm. Hypertrophied foregut endoderm secretes **vascular endothelial growth factor (VEGF),** which induces the sheet of mesoderm to form discontinuous vascular channels that eventually get remodeled into a single **endocardial tube (endocardium).** Mesoderm around the endocardium forms the **myocardium,** which secretes a layer of extracellular matrix proteins called **cardiac jelly.** Mesoderm migrating into the cardiac region from the coelomic wall near the primordial liver forms the **epicardium.**

[handwritten margin note: pericardium = mesoderm, endocardium, myocardium, epicardium]

II Primitive Heart Tube Dilatations *(Figure 1-1E)*

Five dilatations soon become apparent along the length of the tube: the: **truncus arteriosus, bulbus cordis, primitive ventricle, primitive atrium,** and **sinus venosus.** These five dilatations develop into the adult structures of the heart.

III Dextral Looping *(Figure 1-1F and G)*

In the primitive heart tube, venous blood flows through the left ventricle before it flows through the right ventricle. This situation must be corrected because in the normal adult heart venous blood flows into the right ventricle. Dextral looping is the key event in this correction such that the location of the atrioventricular (AV) canal and the conoventricular canal become properly aligned.

A. **Early looping** seems to be inherently programmed within the myocardial cells.

B. **Convergence** begins to bring the AV canal and the conoventricular canal into proper alignment.

C. **Wedging** causes the conoventricular canal to nestle between the tricuspid and mitral valves and occurs concurrently with the formation of the aorticopulmonary (AP) septum.

D. **Repositioning** causes the AV canal to straddle both the right and left ventricles.

IV Partitioning of the Heart Tube

It is important to realize that the primitive heart tube with its five dilatations is a tube with a single lumen, which must be partitioned into four chambers. This partitioning is accomplished by the formation of four septae that divide the single lumen into four chambers. The formation of the four septae are discussed below.

V The Aorticopulmonary (AP) Septum *(Figure 1-2)*

A. **Formation.** Neural crest cells migrate from the hindbrain region through pharyngeal arches 3, 4, and 6 and invade both the **truncal ridges** and **bulbar ridges.** The truncal

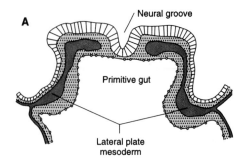

A

Neural groove

Primitive gut

Lateral plate
mesoderm

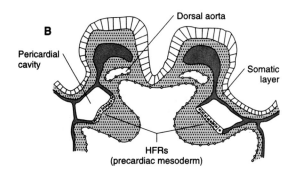

B

Dorsal aorta

Pericardial
cavity

Somatic
layer

HFRs
(precardiac mesoderm)

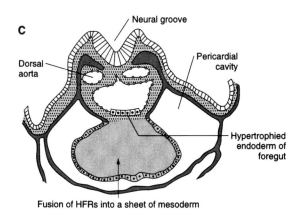

C

Neural groove

Dorsal
aorta

Pericardial
cavity

Hypertrophied
endoderm of
foregut

Fusion of HFRs into a sheet of mesoderm

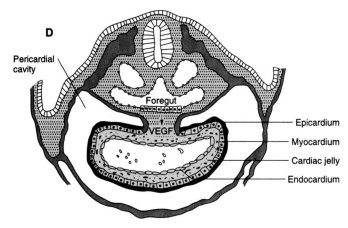

D

Pericardial
cavity

Foregut

VEGF

Epicardium

Myocardium

Cardiac jelly

Endocardium

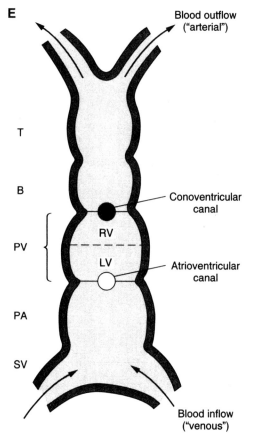

E

Blood outflow
("arterial")

T

B

PV

PA

SV

RV

LV

Conoventricular
canal

Atrioventricular
canal

Blood inflow
("venous")

Embryonic Dilatation	Adult Structure
Truncus arteriosus (T)	Aorta Pulmonary trunk
Bulbus cordis (B)	Smooth part of right ventricle (conus arteriosus) Smooth part of left ventricle (aortic vestibule)
Primitive ventricle (PV)	Trabeculated part of right ventricle (RV) Trabeculated part of left ventricle (LV)
Primitive atrium (PA)	Trabeculated part of right atrium Trabeculated part of left atrium
Sinus venosus (SV)	Smooth part of right atrium (sinus venarum)[a] Coronary sinus Oblique vein of left atrium

[a] The smooth part of the left atrium is formed by incorporation of the transient common pulmonary vein into the atrial wall. The junction of the trabeculated and smooth parts of the right atrium is called the crista terminalis.

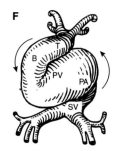

F

T
B
PV
PA
SV

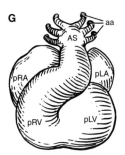

G

aa
AS
pRA
pLA
pRV
pLV

and bulbar ridges grow and twist around each other in a spiral fashion and eventually fuse to form the AP septum. The AP septum divides the truncus arteriosus and bulbus cordis into the aorta and pulmonary trunk.

B. Clinical considerations

1. **Persistent truncus arteriosus (PTA)** is caused by abnormal neural crest cell migration such that there is only *partial* development of the AP septum. PTA results in a condition in which a single arterial vessel with a single semilunar valve arises from the base of the heart and receives blood from both the right and the left ventricles. In **Type I PTA**, a short pulmonary trunk arises from the truncus arteriosus and gives rise to the right and left pulmonary arteries. In **Type II PTA**, the right and left pulmonary arteries arise close to one another directly from the truncus arteriosus. In **Type III PTA**, the right and left pulmonary arteries arise at some distance from one another directly from the truncus arteriosus. PTA is usually accompanied by a membranous ventricular septal defect (VSD) and is associated clinically with **R→L shunting of blood and marked cyanosis**.

2. **D-Transposition of the great arteries (TGA; complete)** is caused by abnormal neural crest cell migration such that there is *non-spiral* development of the AP septum. D-Transposition results in a condition in which the right atrium is connected to the morphological right ventricle by the tricuspid valve, which in turn is discordantly connected to the transposed aorta, and the left atrium is connected to the morphological left ventricle by the mitral valve, which in turn is discordantly connected to the transposed pulmonary trunk. Hence, the systemic and pulmonary circulations are *completely* separated from each other. It is incompatible with life unless an accompanying shunt exists like a VSD, patent foramen ovale, or patent ductus arteriosus (PDA). It is associated clinically with **R→L shunting of blood and marked cyanosis**.

3. **L-Transposition of the great vessels (corrected).** L-Transposition results in a condition in which the right atrium is connected to the morphological left ventricle by the mitral valve, which in turn is discordantly connected to the transposed pulmonary trunk. The left atrium is connected to the morphological right ventricle by the tricuspid valve, which in turn is discordantly connected to the transposed aorta. These two major deviations offset one another such that blood flow pattern is normal.

4. **Double-outlet right ventricle (DORV or incomplete transposition).** In DORV, the aorta and pulmonary trunk both arise primarily from the right ventricle. DORV is usually associated with a VSD that provides the only outlet for blood in the left ventricle. When the VSD is located just beneath the pulmonary semilunar valve, it is called the **Taussig-Bing complex.** DORV is associated clinically with **R→L shunting of blood and marked cyanosis.**

5. **Tetralogy of Fallot (TF)** is caused by an abnormal neural crest cell migration such that there is *skewed* development of the AP septum. TF results in a condition in which the pulmonary trunk obtains a small diameter whereas the aorta obtains a large diameter. TF is characterized by four classic malformations: **pulmonary stenosis, right ventricular hypertrophy, overriding aorta, ventricular septal defect (VSD).** Note the mnemonic **PROVE**. TF is associated clinically with **R→L shunting of blood and marked cyanosis** whereby the clinical consequences

◀

FIGURE 1-1. (A–D) Cross-sections of an embryo at the level of the developing heart. (A) Formation of lateral plate mesoderm. **(B)** Splitting of lateral plate mesoderm. **(C)** Fusion of heart-forming regions (*HFRs*) in the midline into a sheet of mesoderm. **(D)** Vascular endothelial growth factor (*VEGF*) induction of single endocardial tube. **(E–G) Primitive heart tube and its five dilatations. (E) 22 days.** Note the location of the atrioventricular canal and conoventricular canal. Arrows show the direction of blood flow from the "venous" blood inflow at the sinus venosus to the "arterial" blood outflow at the truncus arteriosus. Note that "venous" blood inflow enters the left ventricle (*LV*) before it enters the right ventricle (*RV*). The table indicates the adult structures derived from each embryonic dilatation. **(F) 26 days.** Note that the straight heart tube begins dextral looping (*curved arrows*). B—bulbus cordis; PA—primitive atrium; PV—primitive ventricle; SV—sinus venosus; T—truncus arteriosus. **(G) 30–35 days.** Dextral looping is complete, and the four primitive heart chambers are apparent. aa—aortic arches; AS—aortic sac; pLA—primitive left atrium; pLV—primitive left ventricle; pRA—primitive right atrium; pRV—primitive right ventricle.

depend primarily on the severity of the pulmonary stenosis. In TF, pulmonary blood flow in the neonate depends on a patent ductus arteriosus. The neonate is treated with **prostaglandin infusion (PGE₁)** to maintain the patency of the ductus arteriosus, and a **modified Blalock-Taussig** shunt is surgically placed. A modified Blalock-Taussig shunt is a Gore-Tex shunt placed between the subclavian artery and the pulmonary artery. TF is the most common cyanotic heart malformation and is amenable to surgical repair with good long-term outcomes.

6. **Valvular aortic stenosis (VAS)** is caused by thickening and increased rigidity of valve tissue with varying degrees of commisural separation such that fusion of the cusps of the semilunar valve occurs. Most commonly, the aortic valve is bicuspid with an eccentrically placed orifice. This results in a condition in which the left ventricular blood outflow may be severely restricted. Severe valvular aortic stenosis, aortic hypoplasia, and valvular atresia are components of **hypoplastic left heart syndrome (HLHS)**.

Ⅵ The Atrial Septum *(Figure 1-3)*

A. **Formation.** The crescent-shaped **septum primum** (forms the valve of the fossa ovalis in the adult) develops in the roof of the primitive atrium and grows toward the AV cushions in the AV canal. The **foramen primum** forms between the free edge of the septum primum and the AV cushions and is closed when tissue from the AV septum fuses with the septum primum. The **foramen secundum** forms in the center of the septum primum. The crescent-shaped **septum secundum** (forms the limbus of the fossa ovalis in the adult) develops to the right of the septum primum. The **foramen ovale** is the opening between the upper and lower limbs of the septum secundum. During embryonic life, blood is shunted from the right atrium to the left atrium via the foramen ovale. Immediately after birth, functional closure of the foramen ovale is facilitated both by a **decrease in right atrial pressure** from occlusion of placental circulation and by an **increase in left atrial pressure** due to increased pulmonary venous return whereby the valve of the fossa ovalis is pressed against the limbus to form a competent seal. During the first year of life, the valve and limbus fuse anatomically to produce a permanent seal and an imperforate atrial septum.

B. **Clinical considerations: atrial septal defects (ASDs)**
   1. **Foramen secundum defect** is caused by excessive resorption of septum primum, septum secundum, or both. This results in a condition in an opening between the right and left atria. Some defects can be tolerated for a long time, with clinical symptoms manifesting as late as age 30. The foramen secundum defect is the most common clinically significant ASD. Most infants with ASDs are asymptomatic, but at 6–8 weeks of age a soft systolic murmur along with a fixed and widely split S₂ may be present. ASDs are associated with a **L→ R shunting of blood, fatigue, and dyspnea.**
   2. **Common atrium (cor triloculare biventriculare)** is caused by the complete failure of septum primum and septum secundum to develop. This results in the formation of only one atrium.
   3. **Probe patency of the foramen ovale** is caused by incomplete anatomic fusion of septum primum and septum secundum. It is present in approximately 25% of the population and is usually of no clinical importance.
   4. **Premature closure of foramen ovale** is closure of foramen ovale during prenatal life. It results in hypertrophy of the right side of the heart and underdevelopment of the left side of the heart.

▶

FIGURE 1-2. (A) Formation of the AP septum (*1, 2, 3*). (B) AP septal defects. (a) Persistent truncus arteriosus. (b) D-Transposition of the great arteries (complete). (c) L-Transposition of the great arteries. (d) Double-outlet right ventricle (*DORV*). (e) Tetralogy of Fallot. (f) Aortic valve stenosis with hypoplastic left heart syndrome (*HLHS*). Arrows indicate direction of blood flow. AP—aorticopulmonary; A—aorta; B—bulbus cordis; IV—interventricular; IVC—inferior vena cava; LA—left atrium; LV—left ventricle; PT—pulmonary trunk; RA—right atrium; RV—right ventricle; SVC—superior vena cava; T—truncus arteriosus.

A. Formation of AP Septum

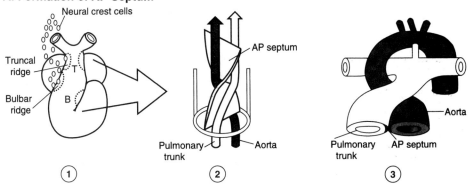

B. AP Septal Defects

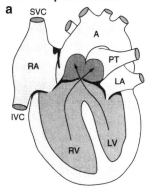

Persistent truncus arteriosus

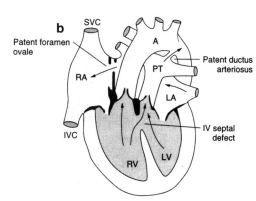

D–Transposition (complete)

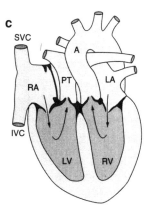

L–Transposition (corrected)

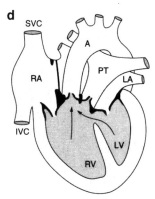

DORV (incomplete)

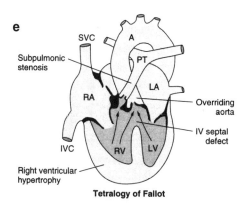

Tetralogy of Fallot

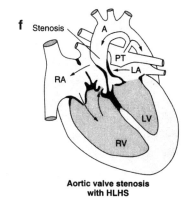

Aortic valve stenosis with HLHS

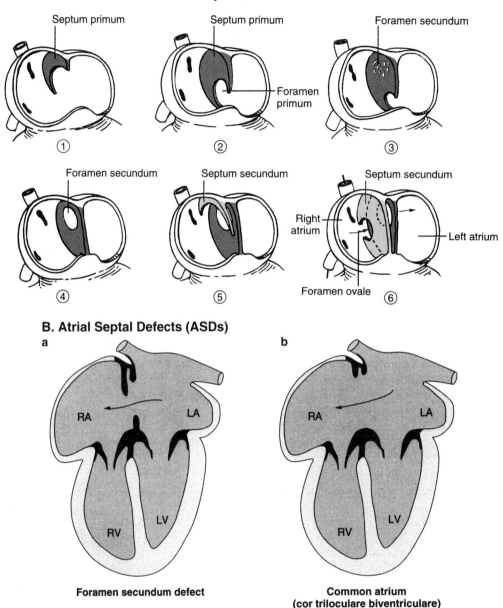

A. Formation of the Atrial Septum

FIGURE 1-3. **(A) Formation of the atrial septum (1–6).** The arrows in 6 indicate the direction of blood flow across the fully developed septum, from the right atrium to the left atrium. **(B) Atrial septal defects. (a) Foramen secundum defect. (b) Common atrium (cor triloculare biventriculare).** Arrows indicate direction of blood flow. LA—left atrium; LV—left ventricle; RA—right atrium; RV—right ventricle.

FIGURE 1-4. **(A) Formation of the AV septum (1, 2, 3,)** which partitions the atrioventricular canal. **(B) AV septal defects. (a) Persistent common AV canal. (b) Foramen primum defect. (c) Ebstein's anomaly. (d) Univentricular heart: double inlet, single inlet, common inlet. (e) Tricuspid atresia.** Arrows indicate direction of blood flow. A—atrium; AV—atrioventricular; Ar—aorta; LA—left atrium; LV—left ventricle; PT—pulmonary trunk; RA—right atrium; RV—right ventricle; V—ventricle.

A. Formation of AV Septum

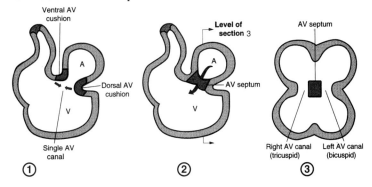

① ② ③

B. AV Septal Defects

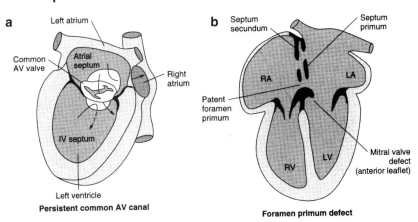

a

Persistent common AV canal

b

Foramen primum defect

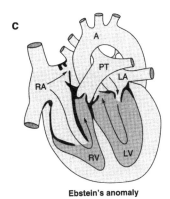

c

Ebstein's anomaly

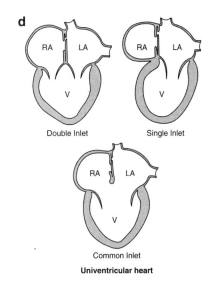

d

Double Inlet   Single Inlet

Common Inlet

Univentricular heart

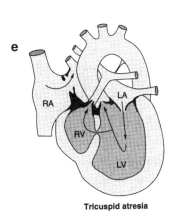

e

Tricuspid atresia

The Atrioventricular Septum (*Figure 1-4*)

A. Formation. The **dorsal AV cushion** and **ventral AV cushion** approach each other and fuse to form the AV septum. The AV septum partitions the AV canal into the right AV canal and left AV canal.

B. Clinical considerations
1. **Persistent common AV canal (complete AV canal)** is caused by failure of fusion of the dorsal and ventral AV cushions. It results in a condition in which the common AV canal is never partitioned into the right and left AV canals so that a large hole can be found in the center of the heart. Consequently, the tricuspid and bicuspid valves are represented by one valve with five leaflets common to both sides of the heart. Two common hemodynamic abnormalities are found:
   a. **L→R shunting of blood** from the left atrium to the right atrium causing an enlarged right atrium and right ventricle
   b. Mitral valve regurgitation causing an enlarged left atrium and left ventricle
2. **Foramen primum defect** is caused by a failure of the AV septum to fuse with the septum primum. It results in a condition in which the foramen primum is never closed and is generally accompanied by an abnormal mitral valve. It is associated clinically with a **L→R shunting of blood.**
3. **Ebstein anomaly** is caused by the failure of the posterior and septal leaflets of the tricuspid valve to attach normally to the annulus fibrosus but are instead displaced inferiorly into the right ventricle. It results in a condition in which the right ventricle is divided into a large, upper, "atrialized" portion **(atrialized right ventricle)** and a small, lower, functional portion **(residual right ventricle).** Owing to the residual right ventricle, a reduced amount of blood is available to the pulmonary trunk. Ebstein anomaly is usually associated with an ASD.
4. **Univentricular heart** is caused by an extremely skewed development of the AV septum to the right and results in a heart with one ventricle. There are three types of univentricular heart: **double-inlet univentricular heart** (most common) occurs when one ventricle receives both the tricuspid and mitral valves; **single-inlet univentricular heart** occurs when one ventricle receives either the tricuspid valve from the left atrium or mitral valve from the right atrium; **common-inlet univentricular heart** occurs when one ventricle receives a common AV valve from the right and left atria. Univentricular heart is usually associated with a VSD.
5. **Tricuspid atresia (TA; hypoplastic right heart)** is caused by an insufficient amount of AV cushion tissue available for the formation of the tricuspid valve. It results in a condition in which there is complete agenesis of the tricuspid valve so that no communication between the right atrium and right ventricle exists. It is associated clinically with **R→L shunting of blood and marked cyanosis** and is always accompanied by the following: patent foramen ovale, interventricular (IV) septum defect, overdeveloped left ventricle, and underdeveloped right ventricle. In Type I TA, the TA is accompanied by normally related great arteries; that is, the aorta is connected to the left ventricle and the pulmonary trunk is connected to the right ventricle. In Type II TA, the TA is accompanied by D-transposition of the great arteries.

VIII The Interventricular (IV) Septum (*Figure 1-5*)

A. Formation. The **muscular IV septum** develops in the midline on the floor of the primitive ventricle and grows toward the fused AV cushions. The **IV foramen** is located between the free edge of the muscular IV septum and the fused AV cushions. This foramen is closed by the **membranous IV septum,** which forms by the proliferation and fusion of tissue from three sources: the **right bulbar ridge, left bulbar ridge,** and **AV cushions.**

B. Clinical considerations: IV septal defects (VSDs)

1. **Membranous VSD** is caused by faulty fusion of the **right bulbar ridge, left bulbar ridge**, and **AV cushions.** The opening between the right and left ventricles is located beneath the aortic semilunar valve (when viewed from the left ventricle) and beneath the supraventricular crest (when viewed from the right ventricle). A large VSD is initially associated with a **L→R shunting of blood**, increased pulmonary blood flow, and pulmonary hypertension. One of the secondary effects of a large VSD and its associated pulmonary hypertension is proliferation of the tunica intima and tunica media of pulmonary muscular arteries and arterioles resulting in a narrowing of their lumen. Ultimately, pulmonary resistance may become higher than systemic resistance and cause **R→L shunting of blood** and cyanosis. At this stage, the characteristic of the patient has been termed the **Eisenmenger complex.** This is the most common type of VSD.

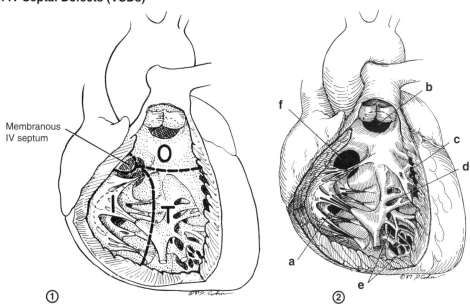

A. Formation of IV Septum

Aorticopulmonary septum

Interventricular foramen

Muscular interventricular septum

Right atrioventricular canal

①

Membranous interventricular septum

Right atrioventricular canal

a b c

Muscular interventricular septum

②

B. IV Septal Defects (VSDs)

Membranous IV septum

O

I T

①

f

b

c

d

a

e

②

FIGURE 1-5. (A) Formation of the interventricular (IV) septum (1, 2) which partitions the primitive ventricle. Shaded portion (a, b, c) in 2 indicates the three sources of the membranous interventricular septum. a—right bulbar ridge; b—left bulbar ridge; c—AV cushions. **(B) IV septal defects. (1)** The IV septum when viewed from the right can be divided into four components: the inlet muscular component (I), outlet muscular component (O), trabecular muscular component (T), and the membranous IV septum. SC—supraventricular crest. **(2)** Diagram shows the anatomical locations of the various VSDs. a—inlet muscular VSD; b—outlet muscular VSD; c—marginal muscular VSD; d—central muscular VSD; e—apical muscular VSD; f—membranous VSD.

2. **Muscular VSDs** are caused by single or multiple perforations in the muscular IV septum and have been categorized based on the location of the perforations as: **an inlet muscular VSD, outlet muscular VSD, marginal muscular VSD, central muscular VSD,** and **apical muscular VSD.**

3. **Common ventricle (cor triloculare biatriatum)** is caused by failure of the membranous and muscular IV septa to form.

Ⓧ Cardiac Malposition

Cardiac malposition describes an abnormal position of the heart as a whole and is usually associated with situs inversus or situs ambiguous. **Situs inversus** describes a right-to-left reversal of viscera. **Situs ambiguous** describes an uncertain position of viscera. **Situs solitus** describes normally positioned viscera.

A. **Dextrocardia with situs solitus (isolated dextrocardia)** is an abnormally positioned heart on the right side of the thorax with the apex pointing to the right and normally positioned viscera. It is usually associated with other severe cardiac abnormalities.

B. **Dextrocardia with situs inversus or situs ambiguous** is an abnormally positioned heart on the right side of the thorax with the apex pointing to the right and either a reversal of viscera (situs inversus) or an uncertain position of viscera (situs ambiguous). It is not usually associated with other severe cardiac abnormalities.

C. **Mesocardia** is an abnormally positioned heart in the midline of the thorax.

D. **Levocardia** is a normally positioned heart on the left side of the thorax with the apex pointing to the left and either a reversal of viscera (situs inversus) or an uncertain position of viscera (situs ambiguous). Levocardia is a term used only in conjunction with situs inversus or situs ambiguous.

Ⓧ The Conduction System of the Heart

At week 5, cardiac myocytes in the sinus venosus region of the primitive heart tube begin to undergo spontaneous electrical depolarizations at a *faster rate* than cardiac myocytes in other regions. As dextral looping occurs, the sinus venous becomes incorporated into the right atrium, and these fast rate depolarizing cardiac myocytes become the **sinoatrial (SA) node** and the **AV node.** In the adult, the cardiac myocytes of the SA and AV nodes remain in an early primitive state committed to fast rate of electrical depolarizations rather than developing contractile properties. As the atria and ventricles become electrically isolated by the formation of the **fibrous skeleton** of the heart, the **AV node** provides the only pathway for depolarizations to flow from the atria to ventricles. The **AV bundle or bundle of His** develops from the **GLN ring,** which is a ringlike cluster of cells found at the AV junction that specifically expresses the **homeobox *msx*-2 gene** and stains specifically with the monoclonal antibody called GLN (ganglion nodosum of the chick). The **intramural network of Purkinje myocytes** have a distinct embryological origin (versus the bundle of His) in that Purkinje myocytes develop from already contractile cardiac myocytes within the myocardium and can therefore be considered as **modified cardiac myocytes.**

Ⓧ Coronary Arteries

A. **General features.** Progenitor stem cells from the liver migrate into the primitive heart tube and take residence beneath the epicardium. These progenitor stem cells invade the future myocardium and form an early **coronary vascular plexus.** The coronary vascular plexus grows toward the truncus arteriosus (future aorta) and forms a **peritruncal capillary ring.** Only two of these capillaries survive, and these become the proximal portions of the right and left coronary arteries.

B. Clinical considerations

1. **Abnormal origin of the left circumflex artery from the right coronary artery.** The left circumflex artery arises abnormally from the right coronary artery (rather than the left coronary artery) and then passes posterior to the aorta to reach its normal territory of supply. This is the most common coronary artery anomaly and generally has no clinical significance.

2. **Abnormal origin of the left coronary artery from the right aortic sinus.** The left coronary artery arises abnormally from the right aortic sinus (rather than the left aortic sinus) whereby the opening of the left coronary artery is slitlike, adheres to the aorta for some distance, and then passes between the pulmonary trunk and ascending aorta. This is not a common anomaly but is associated with sudden death in children during or just after exercise.

3. **Single coronary artery.** A single coronary artery may arise from either the right or left aortic sinus and then branch with many variations to supply the heart. This anomaly is usually associated with other serious heart defects.

XII Development of the Arterial System *(Figure 1-6)*

A. **General pattern.** In the head and neck region, the arterial pattern develops mainly from six pairs of arteries (called **aortic arches**) that course through the pharyngeal arches. The aortic arch arteries undergo a complex remodeling process that results in the adult arterial pattern. In the rest of the body, the arterial pattern develops mainly from the **right and left dorsal aortas.** The right and left dorsal aortas fuse to form the **dorsal aorta,** which then sprouts **posterolateral arteries, lateral arteries,** and **ventral arteries (vitelline and umbilical).**

B. **Clinical considerations.** Most anomalies of the great arteries occur as a result of persistence of parts of the aortic arch system that normally regress and regression of parts that normally persist.

1. **Abnormal origin of the right subclavian artery** occurs when right aortic arch 4 and the right dorsal aorta cranial to the seventh intersegmental artery abnormally regress. As development continues, the right subclavian artery comes to lie on the left side just inferior to the left subclavian artery. The artery must cross the midline posterior to the trachea and esophagus to supply the right arm. This anomaly may constrict the trachea or esophagus. However, it is generally not clinically significant.

2. **Double aortic arch** occurs when an abnormal right aortic arch develops in addition to the left aortic arch owing to persistence of the right and left fourth aortic arches along with the right and left dorsal aortas. This forms a vascular ring around the trachea and esophagus, which causes difficulties in breathing and swallowing.

3. **Right aortic arch with mirror-image branching** occurs when the entire right dorsal aorta abnormally persists and the left dorsal aorta distal to the origin of the seventh intersegmental artery regresses. The first branch off the mirror-image right arch is the left brachiocephalic artery, which divides into the left common carotid and left subclavian arteries; the second branch is the right common carotid artery; and the third branch is the right subclavian artery. The right aortic arch may pass anterior or posterior (retroesophageal right arch) to the esophagus and trachea. A retroesophageal right arch may cause difficulties in swallowing or breathing.

4. **Patent ductus arteriosus (PDA)** occurs when the ductus arteriosus, a connection between the left pulmonary artery and descending aorta fails to close. The ductus arteriosus closes in two phases. In phase 1, smooth muscle contraction and thickening of the tunica media cause the tunica intima to protrude into the lumen resulting in functional closure **within 12 hours after birth.** In phase 2, the smooth muscle of the tunica media is replaced by connective tissue to form the **ligamentum arteriosum within 2–3 weeks after birth.** A PDA causes a **L→R shunting** of oxygen-rich blood

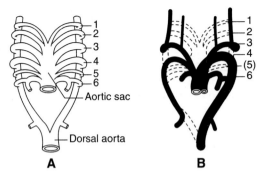

EMBRYONIC	ADULT
Aortic Arch Arteries	
1	Maxillary artery (portion of)
2	Stapedial artery (portion of)
3	R&L common carotid arteries (portion of)
	R&L internal carotid arteries
4	Right subclavian artery (portion of)
	Arch of the aorta (portion of)
5	Regresses in the human
6[a]	R&L pulmonary arteries (portion of)
	Ductus arteriosus
Dorsal Aorta	
Posterolateral arteries	Arteries to the upper and lower extremities, intercostal, lumbar, and lateral sacral arteries
Lateral arteries	Renal, suprarenal, and gonadal arteries
Ventral arteries	
Vitelline	Celiac, superior mesenteric, and inferior mesenteric arteries
	Internal iliac (portion of) and superior vesical arteries
Umbilical	Medial umbilical ligaments

[a]Early in development, the recurrent laryngeal nerves hook around aortic arch 6. On the right side, the distal part of aortic arch 6 regresses, and the right recurrent laryngeal nerve moves up to hook around the right subclavian artery. On the left side, aortic arch 6 persists as the ductus arteriosus (or ligamentum arteriosus in the adult); the left recurrent laryngeal nerve remains hooked around the ductus arteriosus.

D. Clinical Considerations

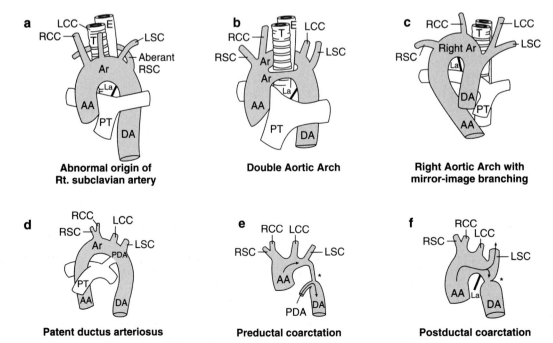

from the aorta back into the pulmonary circulation. **PGE₁, PGE₂, PGI₂,** intrauterine asphyxia, and neonatal asphyxia sustain patency of the ductus arteriosus. **Prostaglandin synthesis inhibitors** (e.g., indomethacin), acetylcholine, histamine, and catecholamines promote closure of the ductus arteriosus. PDA is very common in premature infants, low-birth-weight infants, and maternal rubella infection.

5. **Preductal coarctation (infantile coarctation; isthmic; diffuse-type; less common)** of the aorta occurs when the aorta is abnormally constricted. A preductal coarctation is found distal to the origin of the left subclavian artery and superior to the ductus arteriosus. A preductal coarctation usually has a long segment of aortic narrowing, and a PDA is always present.

6. **Postductal coarctation (adult-type; juxtaductal; discrete-type; most common)** of the aorta occurs when the aorta is abnormally constricted. A postductal coarctation is found distal to the origin of the left subclavian artery and inferior to the ductus arteriosus. It is clinically associated with: increased blood pressure in the upper extremities, diminished and delayed femoral artery pulse, high risk of both cerebral hemorrhage and bacterial endocarditis, rib notching, and Turner's syndrome.

XIII Development of the Venous System *(Figure 1-7)*

A. **General pattern.** The general pattern develops mainly from three pairs of veins: the **vitelline veins, umbilical veins,** and **cardinal veins,** which empty blood into the sinus venosus. These veins undergo remodeling owing to a L→ R shunting of venous blood to the right atrium.

B. **Clinical considerations.** Most anomalies of the venous system occur as a result of persistence of the veins on the left side of the body that normally regress during the L→R shunting of blood.

1. **Left superior vena cava (SVC)** occurs when the left anterior and left common cardinal veins persist, forming an SVC on the left side. The right anterior and right common cardinal veins abnormally regress. In most cases, the left SVC drains into the right atrium through the coronary sinus.

2. **Double SVC** occurs when the left anterior and left common cardinal veins persist, forming an SVC on the left side. The right anterior and right common cardinal veins also form an SVC on the right side. In most cases, the left SVC drains into the right atrium through the coronary sinus.

3. **Double inferior vena cava (IVC)** occurs when the left supracardinal vein persists, forming an IVC on the left side below the level of the kidneys.

4. **Absence of the hepatic portion of the IVC** occurs when the right subcardinal vein fails to form a segment of the IVC. Consequently, blood from the lower part of the body reaches the right atrium via the azygos vein, hemiazygos vein, and SVC.

◄

FIGURE 1-6. (A and B) Development and fate of the aortic arches during the remodeling process. Note the portions of the aortic arches that degenerate during the remodeling process (*dotted lines*). **(C)** Table shows the correspondence of embryonic arteries to their derivative adult counterparts. **(D) Clinical considerations. (a) Abnormal origin of the right subclavian artery. (b) Double aortic arch. (c) Right aortic arch with mirror-image branching. (d) Patent ductus arteriosus. (e) Preductal coarctation.** Blood reaches lower part of the body through a patent ductus arteriosus. Dotted arrows indicate direction of blood flow. Asterisk (*) indicates point of constriction. Prostaglandin treatment is required to maintain the patent ductus arteriosus until surgery. **(f) Postductal coarctation.** Blood reaches lower part of the body via collateral circulation through the left subclavian, intercostal, and internal thoracic arteries. Arrows indicate direction of blood flow. Asterisk (*) indicates point of constriction. AA—ascending aorta; Ar—aortic arch; DA—descending aorta; E—esophagus; LA—ligamentum arteriosum; LCC—left common carotid artery; LSC—left subclavian artery; PDA—patent ductus arteriosus; PT—pulmonary trunk; RCC—right common carotid artery; RSC—right subclavian artery; T—trachea.

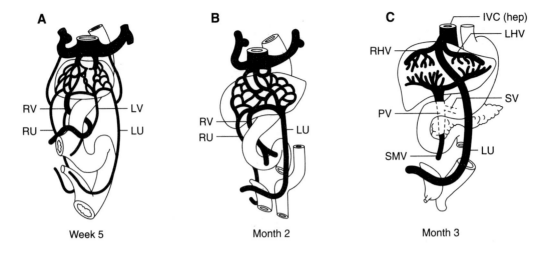

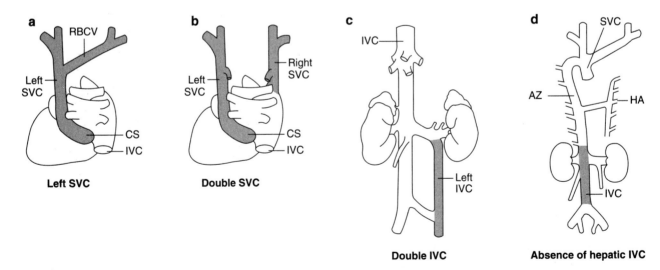

FIGURE 1-7. Development of the vitelline and umbilical veins. (A) Week 5 (B) Month 2 (C) Month 3. Both the vitelline and umbilical veins contribute to the hepatic sinusoidal network within the liver. Owing to the L→R shunting of venous blood, the right vitelline vein enlarges whereas the proximal part of the left vitelline vein disappears. Note that the right umbilical vein degenerates early in fetal life whereas the left umbilical vein enlarges to carry oxygenated blood from the placenta to the fetus. IVC—inferior vena cava; PV—portal vein; RHV—right hepatic vein; RU—right umbilical vein; RV—right vitelline vein; SMV—superior mesenteric vein; SV—splenic vein. **(D)** Table shows the correspondence of the embryonic veins to their adult counterparts. **(E) Clinical considerations. (a) Left SVC. (b) Double SVC. (c) Double IVC. (d) Absence of hepatic portion of the IVC.** AZ—azygos vein; CS—coronary sinus; HA—hemiazygos; RBCV—right brachiocephalic vein.

D.

EMBRYONIC	ADULT
Vitelline Veins	
Right and left	Portion of the IVC, hepatic veins and sinusoids, ductus venosus, portal vein, inferior mesenteric vein, superior mesenteric vein, splenic vein
Umbilical Veins	
Right	Hepatic sinusoids, degenerates early in fetal life
Left	Hepatic sinusoids, ligamentum teres
Cardinal Veins	
Anterior	SVC, internal jugular veins
Posterior	Portion of IVC, common Iliac veins
Subcardinal	Portion of IVC, renal veins, gonadal veins
Supracardinal	Portion of IVC, intercostal veins, hemiazygos vein, azygos vein

IVC — inferior vena cava; SVC — superior vena cava.

Note that the IVC is derived embryologically from four different sources.

E. Clinical Considerations

XIV Development of the Pulmonary Veins *(Figure 1-8)*

A. **Formation.** In the early stages of human development, the lung bud is surrounded by a vascular plexus called the **foregut plexus.** As lung development continues, the foregut plexus forms a **pulmonary vascular bed.** At this stage of development, no direct connection between the lungs and heart exists. Instead, the pulmonary vascular bed shares the same routes of drainage of the foregut plexus into the vitelline, umbilical, and cardinal system of veins. Later in development, the **common pulmonary vein** develops as an outgrowth of the dorsal wall of the left atrium and establishes a connection to the pulmonary vascular bed. When this occurs, the connections between the pulmonary vascular bed and the foregut plexus involute. Consequently, the pulmonary vascular bed drains via **four pulmonary veins** into the common pulmonary vein, which in turn empties into the left atrium. As the left atrium grows, the transient common pulmonary vein is incorporated into the wall of the left atrium, forming the **smooth part of the left atrium.**

B. **Clinical considerations**
   1. **Total anomalous pulmonary venous return** occurs when none of the four pulmonary veins connect to the left atrium but instead drain into a horizontal venous confluence (HVC)→left brachiocephalic vein (BCV)→SVC (Type I). The pulmonary veins may also drain into the coronary sinus or right atrium (Type II) or portal vein (Type III). The presence of an ASD or patent foramen ovale is necessary to sustain life.
   2. **Partial anomalous pulmonary venous return** occurs when the two right pulmonary veins drain into the left atrium but the two left pulmonary veins drain into the left brachiocephalic vein or inferior vena cava. Another configuration occurs when the two right pulmonary veins drain into the inferior vena cava but the two left pulmonary veins drain into the left atrium.

XV Fetal and Neonatal Circulation *(Figure 1-9)*

A. **Fetal circulation.** The **left umbilical vein** carries high O_2-content blood from the placenta to the liver, where 50% of the blood percolates through the **hepatic sinusoids** to the IVC and 50% of the blood enters the **ductus venous** (a fetal shunt that connects the left umbilical vein to the IVC). The **IVC** carries medium O_2-content blood (because the IVC also receives low O_2-content blood from the lower limbs, pelvis, and abdomen via the portal vein) to the **right atrium,** where most of the blood enters the **foramen ovale** (a right-to-left fetal shunt that connects the **right atrium** to the left atrium) and is shunted to the left atrium, which also receives low O_2-content blood from the **pulmonary veins.** The **left ventricle** ejects medium O_2-content blood to the **ascending and descending aorta,** which perfuses the head/neck and rest of the body, respectively. The remainder of the blood from the IVC and the low O_2-content blood from the SVC mixes in the right atrium and enters the **right ventricle.** The **right ventricle** ejects medium O_2-content blood to the **pulmonary trunk,** where 10% of the blood enters the lungs and 90% of the blood enters the **ductus arteriosus.** The ductus arteriosus (a **R→L fetal shunt**) develops from aortic arch 6 and connects the left pulmonary artery with the descending aorta 5–10 mm distal to the left subclavian artery. By week 6 of development, the ductus arteriosus carries most of the right ventricular output. The **descending aorta** carries medium O_2-content blood where 35% of the blood is distributed to the fetal body (and returned to the fetal circulation as low O_2-content blood) and 65% of the blood is returned to the placenta by the **right and left umbilical arteries.**

B. **Neonatal circulation.** At birth, the right and left umbilical arteries, left umbilical vein, ductus venous, ductus arteriosus, and foramen ovale close, cease to function, and form

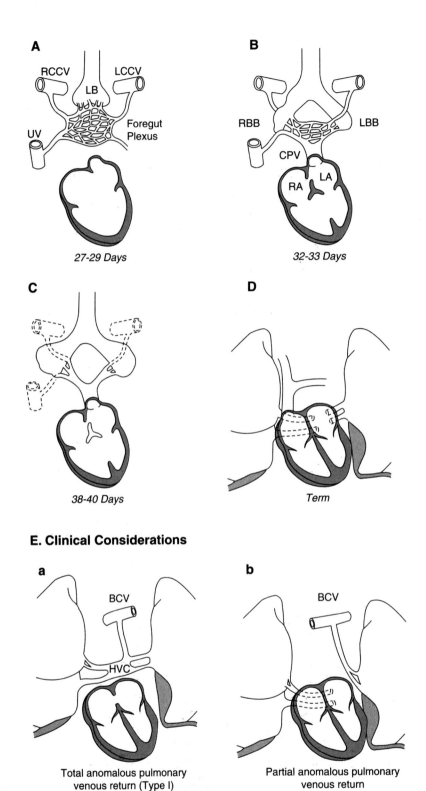

FIGURE 1-8. Development of the pulmonary veins. (A) 27–29 days. The lung bud (*LB*) is surrounded by the foregut plexus, which forms a pulmonary vascular bed. Note that there is no direct connection between the lungs and heart. Instead, the pulmonary vascular bed shares the same routes of drainage of the foregut plexus into the vitelline, umbilical, and cardinal system of veins. LCCV—left common cardinal vein; RCCV—right common cardinal vein; UV—umbilical vein. **(B) 32–33 days.** The common pulmonary vein (*CPV*) establishes a connection between the pulmonary vascular bed and the left atrium (*LA*). RA—right atrium; LBB—left bronchial bud; RBB—right bronchial bud. **(C) 38–40 days.** The connections between the pulmonary vascular bed and the foregut plexus involute. **(D) Term.** The common pulmonary vein is incorporated into the wall so that four pulmonary veins open directly into the left atrium. **(E) Clinical considerations. (a) Type I total anomalous pulmonary venous return.** Note that none of the pulmonary venous blood drains into the left atrium but instead drains into the horizontal venous confluence (*HVC*)→left brachiocephalic vein (*BCV*)→superior vena cava. **(b) Partial anomalous pulmonary venous return.** Note that none of the pulmonary venous blood from the left lung drains into the left atrium but instead drains into the left brachiocephalic vein (*BCV*)→superior vena cava. However, pulmonary venous blood from the right lung drains into the right atrium normally.

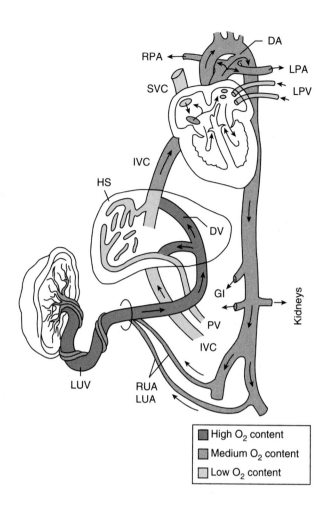

FIGURE 1-9. Diagram of fetal circulation. DA—ductus arteriosus; DV—ductus venous; GI—gastrointestinal tract; HS—hepatic sinusoids; IVC—inferior vena cava; LPA—left pulmonary artery; LPV—left pulmonary veins; LUA—left umbilical artery; LUV—left umbilical vein; PV—portal vein; RPA—right pulmonary artery; RUA—right umbilical artery; SVC—superior vena cava. The table shows the adult remnants created by closure of the fetal structures.

adult remnants. The **right atrial pressure decreases** as a result of the occlusion of the placental circulation. The **left atrial pressure increases** as a result of increased pulmonary return from the lungs. The transition from fetal to neonatal circulation is marked when the fluid-filled lungs are distended with air during the first breath. This induces a **rapid decrease in pulmonary vascular resistance (PVR)** and an **increased pulmonary blood flow.** The PVR is further reduced by the production of vasodilators, in particular, **prostacyclin** and **nitric oxide** by the neonatal lung. Later, the PVR is further reduced by a **progressive thinning of the smooth muscle layer** (tunica media) of pulmonary arterial vasculature.

ⓧⓥⓘ The Pediatric Thorax *(Figure 1-10)*

The chest of a normal newborn infant has a **lamp-shade** or **trapezoidal appearance**, which by 6 years of age approaches the long, thin shape seen in the adult. The **posterior mediastinal line** produced by the right pleuromediastinal reflection and various **pulmonary fissures** are regularly seen radiographically in newborns and infants.

A

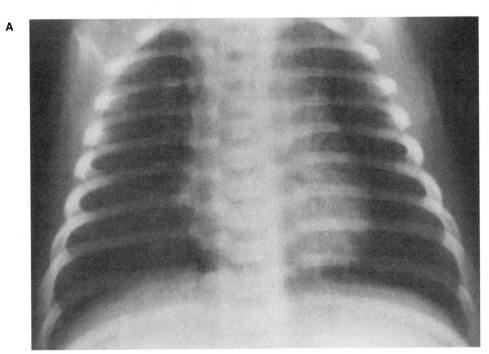

Newborn

B

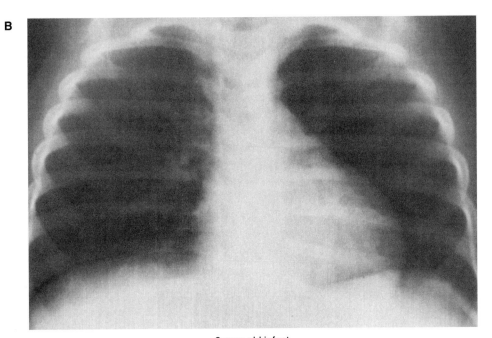

2-year-old infant

FIGURE 1-10. (A–C) Pediatric thorax. (A) AP radiograph shows a lamp-shade or trapezoid appearance of the chest in a normal newborn infant. **(B)** AP radiograph of the chest in a 2-year-old normal infant.

(continued)

C

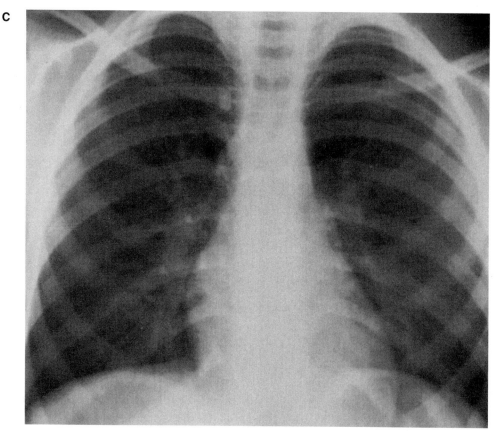

6-year-old child

FIGURE 1-10 *(continued)* **(C)** AP radiograph of the chest in a 6-year-old normal child.

ⅩⅦ Radiographs, Echocardiograms, Angiograms, and Magnetic Resonance Imaging

A. **Aorticopulmonary (AP) septal defects** *(Figure 1-11)*

B. **Atrial septal defects (ASDs)** *(Figure 1-12)*

C. **Atrioventricular (AV) septal defects** *(Figure 1-13)*

D. **Interventricular (IV) septal defects (VSDs)** *(Figure 1-14)*

E. **Cardiac malpositions** *(Figure 1-15)*

F. **Arterial system defects** *(Figure 1-16)*

G. **Venous system defects** *(Figure 1-17)*

H. **Pulmonary vein defects** *(Figure 1-18)*

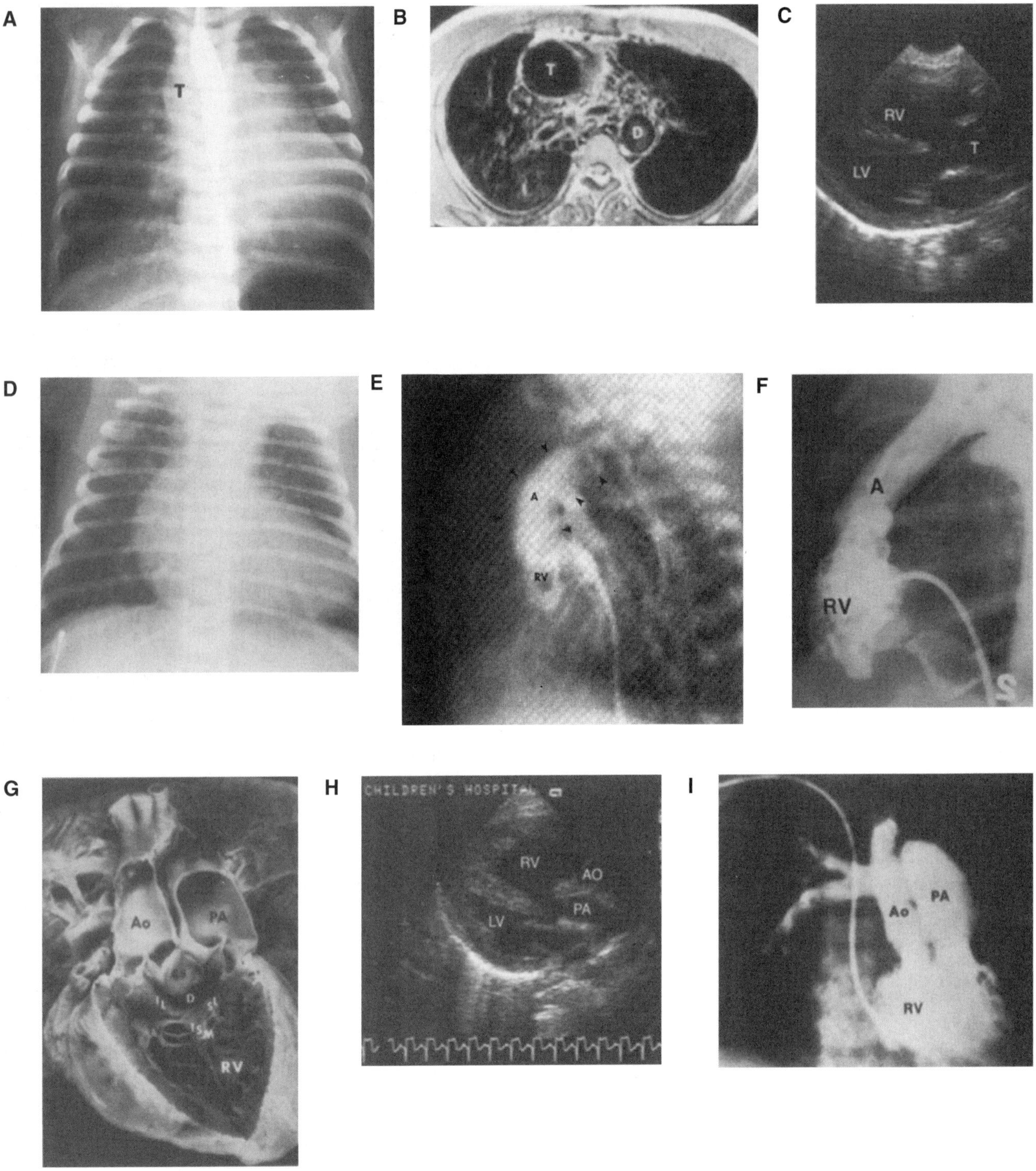
A
B
C
T
T
D
RV
LV
T
D
E
F
A
RV
A
RV
G
H
I
Ao
PA
RV
CHILDREN'S HOSPITAL
RV
AO
LV
PA
Ao
PA
RV

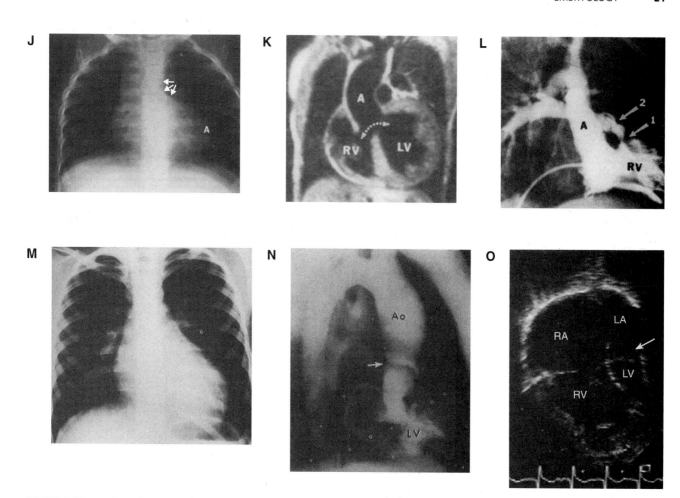

FIGURE 1-11. Aorticopulmonary (AP) septal defects. (A–C) Type I persistent truncus arteriosus (PTA). (A) Radiograph shows cardiomegaly and downward dipping of the heart apex, which suggests left ventricle dilatation. Radiographs of Type II and Type III PTA usually show a typical oval cardiomegaly. Note that the truncus arteriosus (*T*) is on the right. **(B)** Coronal MRI shows a large truncus arteriosus (*T*) and descending aorta (*D*). Note that there is no pulmonary trunk in the normal anatomical position. **(C)** Parasternal long-axis echocardiogram shows the truncus arteriosus (*T*) over-riding the interventricular septum whereby it receives blood from both the right and left ventricles. **(D–F) D-Transposition of the great arteries (TGA; complete). (D)** Radiograph shows an oval or egg-shaped heart with a narrow superior mediastinum due to the abnormal positions of the great vessels (i.e., the aorta and pulmonary trunk lie directly behind each other); absence of the aortic arch along the left border of the heart; absence of the pulmonary trunk along the left border of the heart; asymmetry of pulmonary blood flow to the right because left ventricular ejection into the pulmonary trunk is oriented more toward the right than normal. **(E)** Coronal MRI shows the transposed aorta (*A*) positioned anteriorly and to the right of the pulmonary trunk (*P*). **(F)** Angiogram of the right ventricle shows the aorta (*A*) arising from the right ventricle (*RV*). **(G–I) Double-outlet right ventricle (DORV). (G)** Photograph of gross specimen shows the interior of the right ventricle (*RV*), aorta (*Ao*), and pulmonary trunk (*PA*). Note the side-by-side relationship of the aorta and pulmonary trunk arising from the right ventricle. In a radiograph of DORV, the superior mediastinum is wide because of the side-by-side relationship of the aorta and pulmonary trunk in contrast to transposition of the great arteries where the superior mediastinum is narrow because the aorta and pulmonary trunk lie directly behind each other. The ventricular septal defect (*D*) is cradled between the inferior limb (*IL*) and the superior limb (*SL*) of the trabecula septomarginalis (*TSM*). **(H)** Parasternal long-axis echocardiogram shows the aorta and pulmonary trunk arising from the right ventricle. Note the ventricular septal defect. **(I)** Angiogram shows the aorta and pulmonary trunk arising from the right ventricle. **(J–L) Tetralogy of Fallot. (J)** Radiograph shows a normal-sized heart, an upturned cardiac apex (*A*), concavity at the pulmonary trunk site (*arrows*), and decreased pulmonary arterial blood flow. **(K)** Coronal MRI shows the overriding aorta (*A*) over the right ventricle (*RV*) and left ventricle (*LV*). The ventricular septal defect is indicated by the dotted arrow. **(L)** Angiogram (right anterior oblique view) shows the pulmonary stenosis (*1*) and some thickening of the stenotic pulmonary valve (*2*). **(M–O) Valvular aortic stenosis (VAS). (M)** Radiograph shows a moderately enlarged heart, a rounded cardiac apex, and hypertrophy of the left ventricle. The size of the left ventricle does not correlate closely with the size of the aortic orifice. **(N)** Angiogram shows a thickening of the aortic valve cusps (*arrow*) and poststenotic dilatation of the ascending aorta (*Ao*). **(O)** Parasternal long-axis echocardiogram shows the four-chambered view of a hypoplastic left heart syndrome. Note the small left ventricle (*LV*) and atretic mitral valve (*arrow*). LA—left atrium; RA—right atrium; RV—right ventricle.

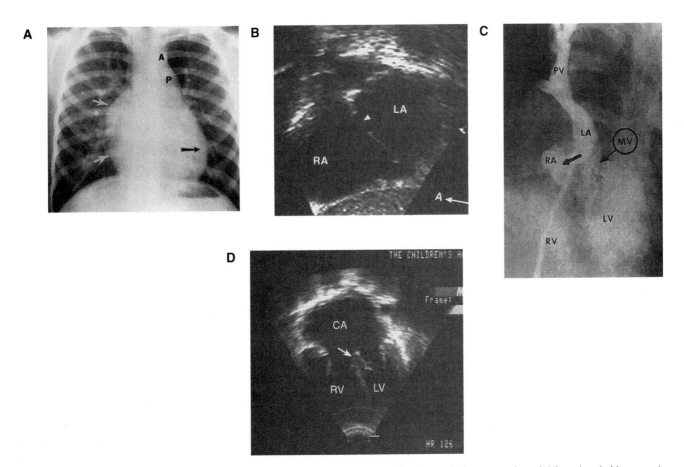

FIGURE 1-12. Atrial septal defects (ASDs). (A–C) Foramen secundum defect. (A) Radiograph shows an enlarged right atrium (*white arrows*), increased pulmonary vascularity, a large pulmonary artery (*P*), a small aorta (*A*), and the cardiac apex pointing laterally (*black arrow*). The L→R shunt leads to increased delivery of blood to the right atrium during systole and diastole, which leads to volume overload and enlargement of the right atrium. Subsequently, the right ventricle and pulmonary artery also enlarge and therefore increase pulmonary vascularity. **(B)** Subcostal short-axis echocardiogram shows a defect in the atrial septum (*arrowhead*) between the left atrium (*LA*) and right atrium (*RA*). **(C)** Angiogram shows contrast material passing from the left atrium (*LA*) to right atrium (*RA*) through an atrial septal defect (*arrow*). The contrast material is injected into a pulmonary vein (*PV*). LV—left ventricle; MV—mitral valve region; RV—right ventricle. **(D) Common atrium (cor triloculare biventriculare).** Apical four-chambered echocardiogram shows a common atrium (*CA*) with no apparent atrial septum. Arrow—atrioventricular (*AV*) septum.

▶

FIGURE 1-13. Atrioventricular (AV) septal defects. (A and B) Persistent common AV canal (complete atrioventricular canal). (A) Radiograph shows an oval-shaped enlarged heart with an enlarged right atrium (*arrows*) and right ventricle. **(B)** Angiogram shows the typical elongated left ventricular outflow tract called the "gooseneck" deformity (*white arrows*). This is caused by a deep excursion of the abnormal mitral valve leaflets into the left ventricle, resulting in an apparent elongation of the left ventricular outflow tract. The deformed mitral valve leaflets may appear bilobed (*black arrows*), irregular, or scalloped. **(C) Foramen primum defect.** Apical four-chambered echocardiogram shows a foramen primum defect (arrow) due to the failure of the AV septum to fuse with septum primum. **(D–F) Ebstein anomaly (D)** Radiograph shows an enlarged heart due to an enormously enlarged right atrium. Note the abnormal left cardiac contour due to the displacement of the right ventricular outflow tract. The pulmonary vascularity is decreased. **(E)** Radiograph shows a box-shaped enlarged heart due to the elevated residual right ventricle seen along the upper left cardiac border (*arrows*) Enlargement of the right atrium is not as conspicuous as in radiograph D. **(F)** Angiogram shows the entire heart opacified due to the general stagnation of circulation in the heart. Note the right atrium (*RA*), atrialized right ventricle (*ARV*), and residual right ventricle (*RV*).1—annulus fibrosis; 2—displaced posterior and septal leaflets of the tricuspid valve. **(G–J) Univentricular heart. (G)** Apical four-chambered echocardiogram shows a double-inlet univentricular heart. L—left; LA—left atrium; MVC—main ventricular chamber; PV—pulmonary valve; R—right; RA—right atrium. **(H and I) Gross specimen and echocardiogram comparison of a single inlet univentricular heart. (H)** Photograph of gross specimen shows a single-inlet univentricular heart. Note the tiny, slitlike remnant of the right ventricle (*arrow*). The arrowhead points to the junction of the atrial septum (*AS*) and interventricular septum (*VS*), which are aligned. The morphological left ventricle (*LV*) with the mitral valve (*MV*) is the main ventricular chamber. LV—left ventricle. **(I)** Apical four-chambered echocardiogram shows a single-inlet univentricular heart. The arrowhead points to the junction of the atrial septum (*AS*) and interventricular septum (*VS*), which are aligned. The main ventricular chamber (*MVC*) is the morphological left ventricle with the left (*L*) atrioventricular valve (mitral valve). **(J)** Apical four-chambered echocardiogram shows a common inlet univentricular heart. AS—atrial septum; CAVV—common atrioventricular valve. **(K and L) Tricuspid atresia (K)** Radiograph shows a normal-sized heart with a convexity of lower left heart border, an elevated apex, a concave pulmonary trunk, and decreased pulmonary vascularity. **(L)** Angiogram shows no forward flow of contrast material from the RA into the right ventricle. Instead, the contrast material passes into the LA through an atrial septal defect (ASD) and then into the LV. A triangular lucency (*arrow*) is found in a position normally occupied by the inflow portion of the right ventricle just to the left of the tricuspid valve.

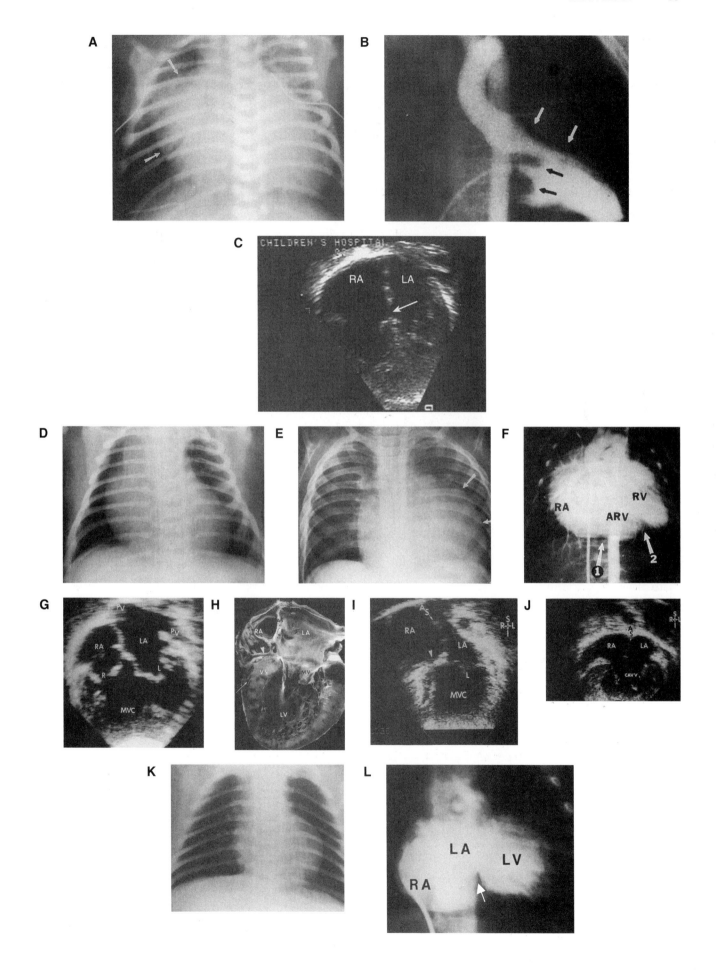

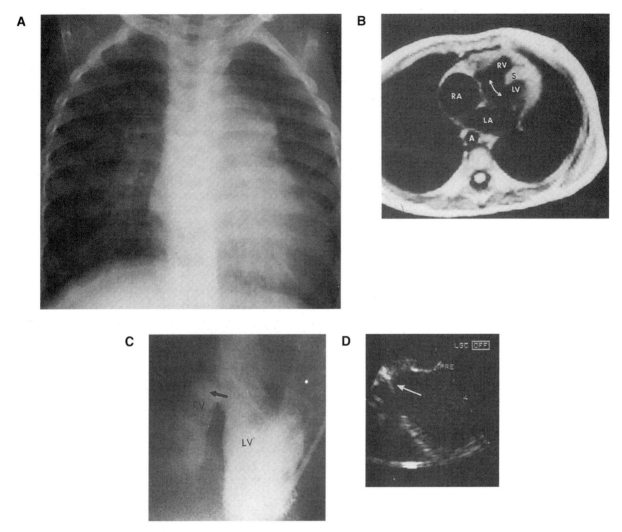

FIGURE 1-14. Interventricular septal defects (VSDs). (A) Radiograph shows an enlarged heart, marked enlargement of the pulmonary trunk, and increased pulmonary vascularity. Left ventricular dilatation produces a dipping or sagging of the cardiac apex, which points downward. **(B)** MRI shows a large interventricular septal defect (*arrow*). A—aorta; LA—left atrium; LV—left ventricle; RA—right atrium; RV—right ventricle; S—interventricular septum. **(C)** Angiogram shows contrast material passing from the left ventricle (*LV*) into the right ventricle (*RV*) through a large high interventricular septal defect in the membranous septum (i.e., a membranous VSD). **(D)** Transesophageal echocardiogram shows an interventricular septal defect in the muscular septum (i.e., muscular VSD). The arrow points to muscular tissue on the superior edge of the defect.

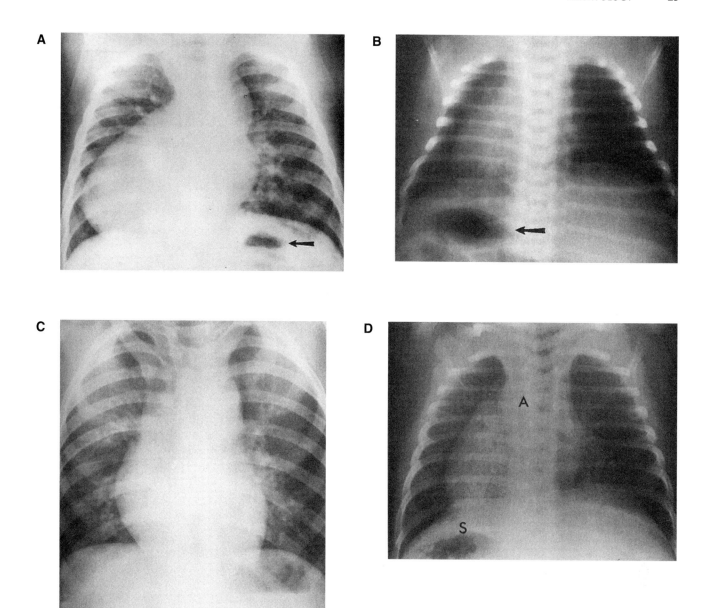

FIGURE 1-15. Cardiac malpositions. (A) Dextrocardia with situs solitus (isolated dextrocardia). Radiograph shows the heart on the right side of the thorax with the cardiac apex pointing to the right. Note that the stomach is on the normal left side indicated by the gastric bubble (*arrow*). **(B) Dextrocardia with situs inversus.** Radiograph shows heart on the right side of the thorax with the cardiac apex pointing to the right. Note that the stomach is on the abnormal right side indicated by the gastric bubble (*arrow*) and the liver is on the left side. **(C) Mesocardia.** Radiograph shows the heart abnormally positioned in the midline of the thorax. **(D) Levocardia.** Radiograph shows the heart on the normal left side of the thorax with the cardiac apex pointing to the left. Note that the stomach (*S*) is on the abnormal right side. A—aorta.

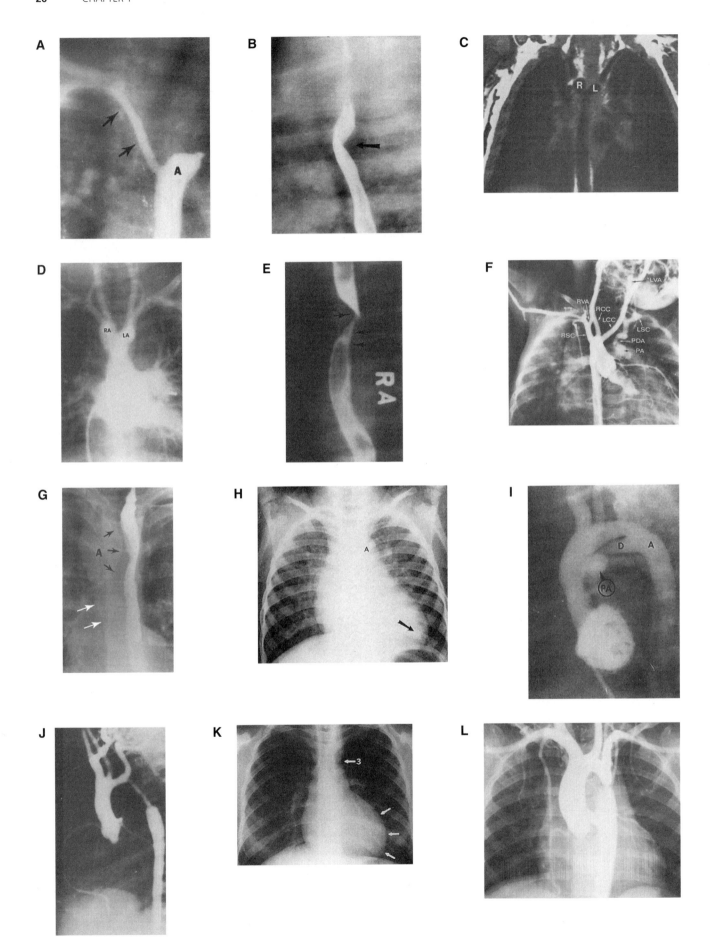

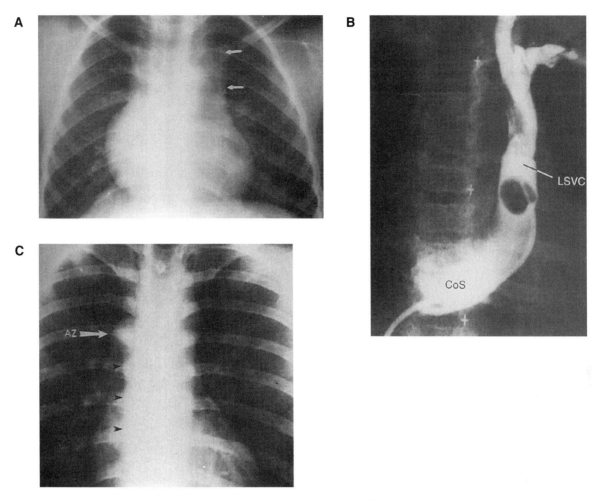

FIGURE 1-17. (A and B) Left superior vena cava. (A) Radiograph shows a widening of the superior mediastinum and an abnormal fullness along the left side (*arrows*). **(B)** Venogram shows a left superior vena cava (*LSVC*) draining into the coronary sinus (*CoS*). Note the absence of a normal right SVC. **(C) Absence of the hepatic portion of the inferior vena cava.** Radiograph shows a characteristic enlargement on the right side of the azygos vein (*AZ*) and an associated paraspinal stripe (*arrowheads*) resulting from continuation of the inferior vena cava into the azygos vein.

◄

FIGURE 1-16. Arterial system defects. (A and B) Abnormal origin of the right subclavian artery. (A) Aortogram shows the characteristic course of the aberrant right subclavian artery (*arrows*). Contrast material was injected into the descending aorta (*A*). **(B)** Barium esophagram (lateral view) shows the characteristic finger-like indentation of the posterior aspect of the esophagus. An aberrant right subclavian artery rarely presents with clinical symptoms and is usually an incidental finding during an upper gastrointestinal examination. However, clinical signs may include: dysphagia, food lodging within the esophagus, and respiratory compromise. **(C and D) Double aortic arch. (D)** Aortogram shows the typical appearance of a double aortic arch. LA—left aortic arch; RA—right aortic arch. **(E)** Barium esophagram (anteroposterior view) shows the reverse S-shaped configuration of the esophagus resulting from the larger, posterior right aortic arch (*upper arrow*) and the smaller, anterior left aortic arch (*lower arrows*). **(F and G) Right aortic arch. (F)** Aortogram shows a right aortic arch with the left common carotid artery (*LCC*), right common carotid artery (*RCC*), and right subclavian artery (*RSC*) branching directly from the arch. This example of right aortic arch has a peculiar branching pattern in that there is no left brachiocephalic artery; instead there is an isolated left subclavian artery (*LSC*) that receives blood from the aorta via retrograde flow from the left vertebral artery (*LVA*) that constitutes the congenital subclavian steal syndrome. Note there is L→R shunting of blood through a patent ductus arteriosus (PDA). PA—pulmonary artery; RVA—right vertebral artery. **(G)** Barium esophagram (anteroposterior view) shows the right aortic arch (*A*). Note the indentation and displacement of the trachea and esophagus (*upper arrows*) and the slanted line (*lower arrows*) indicating the proximal portion of the descending aorta on the right side. **(H and I) Patent ductus arteriosus (PDA). (H)** Radiograph shows an enlarged heart, downward dipping of the cardiac apex (*arrow*) due to left ventricular dilatation, and an enlarged aortic arch or knob (*A*). **(I)** Aortogram shows a moderately long ductus arteriosus (*D*) between the left pulmonary artery (*PA*) and descending aorta (*A*). **(J–L) Coarctation of the aorta. (J) Preductal coarctation.** Aortogram shows a long segment of aortic narrowing distal to the left subclavian artery and superior to the ductus arteriosus. **(K and L) Postductal coarctation. (K)** Radiograph shows a well-rounded appearance of the left heart border (*arrows*) resulting from left ventricular hypertrophy. Note the presence of a "figure 3" sign where the upper bulge represents the prestenotic dilatation and the lower bulge represents the poststenotic dilatation. **(L)** Aortogram shows a discrete aortic narrowing distal to the left subclavian artery and inferior to the ductus arteriosus.

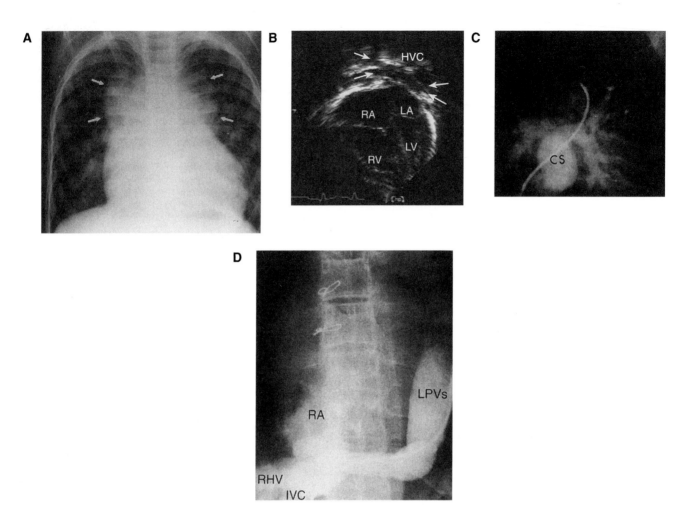

FIGURE 1-18. (A–C) Total anomalous pulmonary venous return. (A and B) Type I total anomalous pulmonary venous return. (A) Radiograph shows the characteristic "snowman" or "figure 8" appearance (*arrows*) due to the horizontal venous confluence located just posterior to the left atrium. Note the enlarged right atrium, enlarge right ventricle, and increased pulmonary vascularity. **(B)** Apical four-chambered echocardiogram shows four pulmonary veins (*arrows*) entering the horizontal venous confluence (*HVC*). Note the reduced size of the left atrium (*LA*) and left ventricle (*LV*). RA—right atrium; RV—right ventricle. **(C) Type II total anomalous pulmonary venous return.** Angiogram shows the pulmonary veins draining directly into the coronary sinus (*CS*). **(D) Partial anomalous pulmonary venous return.** Angiogram shows the left pulmonary veins draining directly into the inferior vena cava (*IVC*). The right pulmonary veins drain normally into the left atrium. RA—right atrium; RHV—right hepatic vein.

Chapter 2

Gross Anatomy

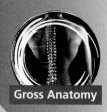

THE THORAX

❶ Bones of the Thorax

A. Thoracic vertebrae. There are 12 thoracic vertebrae that have facets on their bodies (**costal facets**) for articulation with the heads of ribs, facets on their transverse processes for articulation with the tubercles of rib 9 (except for ribs 11 and 12), and long spinous processes.

B. Ribs. There are 12 pairs of ribs that articulate with the thoracic vertebrae. A rib consists of a **head, neck, tubercle, and body.** The head articulates with the body of adjacent thoracic vertebrae and the intervertebral disk at the **costovertebral joint.** The tubercle articulates with the transverse process of a thoracic vertebra at the **costo-transverse joint.**
   1. **True (vertebrosternal) ribs** are **ribs 1–7,** which articulate individually with the sternum by their costal cartilages.
   2. **False (vertebrochondral) ribs** are **ribs 8–12.** Ribs 8–10 articulate with more superior costal cartilage and form the **anterior costal margin.** Ribs 11 and 12 (often called **floating ribs**) articulate with vertebral bodies but do not articulate with the sternum.

C. Sternum consists of the following:
   1. The **manubrium** forms the **jugular notch** at its superior margin, has a **clavicular notch** that articulates with the clavicle at the **sternoclavicular joint,** and articulates with the costal cartilages of ribs 1 and 2.
   2. The **body** articulates with the manubrium at the **sternal angle of Louis,** with the costal cartilages of ribs 2–7, and with the **xiphoid process** at the **xiphosternal joint.**
   3. The **xiphoid process** articulates with the body of the sternum and attaches to the diaphragm and abdominal musculature via the **linea alba.**
   4. The **sternal angle of Louis** marks the junction between the manubrium and the body of the sternum at vertebral level T4. This is the site where: rib 2 articulates with the sternum, the aortic arch begins and ends, the trachea bifurcates, and the superior mediastinum ends.

❷ Muscles of the Thorax

A. The **diaphragm (most important muscle of inspiration)** elevates the ribs and increases the vertical, transverse (bucket-handle movement), and anteroposterior (pump-handle movement) diameters of the thorax. The diaphragm is innervated by the **phrenic nerves** (ventral primary rami of C3-C5), which provide motor and sensory innervation. Sensory innervation to the periphery of the diaphragm is provided by the **intercostal nerves.** A lesion of the phrenic nerve may result in **paralysis** and

paradoxical movement of the diaphragm. The paralyzed dome of the diaphragm does not descend during inspiration and is consequently forced upward because of increased abdominal pressure.

B.   The **intercostal muscles** are thin multiple layers of muscle that occupy the **intercostal spaces (1-11)** and keep the intercostal space rigid during inspiration or expiration. The **external intercostal muscles** elevate the ribs and play a role in inspiration during exercise or lung disease. The **internal intercostal muscles** play a role in expiration during exercise or lung disease. The **innermost intercostal muscles** are presumed to act with the internal intercostal muscles. The intercostal vein, artery, and nerve run between the internal intercostal muscles and innermost intercostal muscles.

C.   The **sternocleidomastoid, pectoralis major** and **minor,** and the **scalene muscles** attach to the ribs and play a role in inspiration during exercise or lung disease.

D.   The **external oblique, internal oblique, transverse abdominus,** and **rectus abdominis muscles** (i.e., abdominal muscles) play a role in expiration during exercise, lung disease, or the Valsalva maneuver.

Ⅲ   Nerves of the Thorax

The **intercostal nerves** are the ventral primary rami of T1-T11 and run in the **costal groove** between the internal intercostal muscles and innermost intercostal muscles. The **subcostal nerve** is the ventral primary ramus of T12. Intercostal nerve injury is evidenced by a sucking in (upon inspiration) and bulging out (upon expiration) of the affected intercostal space.

Ⅳ   Arteries of the Thorax

A.   **Internal thoracic artery** is a branch of the **subclavian artery** that descends just lateral to the sternum and terminates at intercostal space 6 by dividing into the **superior epigastric artery** and **musculophrenic artery.**

B.   **Anterior intercostal arteries.** The anterior intercostal arteries that supply intercostal spaces 1-6 are branches of the **internal thoracic artery.** The anterior intercostal arteries that supply intercostal spaces 7-9 are branches of the **musculophrenic artery.** Two anterior intercostal arteries are within each intercostal space that anastomose with the posterior intercostal arteries.

C.   **Posterior intercostal arteries.** The posterior intercostal arteries that supply intercostal spaces 1-2 are branches of the **superior intercostal artery,** which arises from the **costocervical trunk** of the subclavian artery. The posterior intercostal arteries that supply intercostal spaces 3-11 are branches of the **thoracic aorta.** The **subcostal artery** is also a branch of the thoracic aorta. All posterior intercostal arteries give off a posterior branch, which travels with the dorsal primary ramus of a spinal nerve to supply the spinal cord, vertebral column, back muscles, and skin. The posterior intercostal arteries anastomose anteriorly with the anterior intercostal arteries.

Ⅴ   Veins of the Thorax

A.   **Anterior intercostal veins.** The anterior intercostal veins drain the anterior thorax and empty into the **internal thoracic veins,** which then empty into the **brachiocephalic veins.**

B. **Posterior intercostal veins.** The posterior intercostal veins drain the lateral and posterior thorax and empty into the **hemiazygos veins** on the left side and the **azygos vein** on the right side. The hemiazygos veins empty into the azygos vein, which empties into the superior vena cava (SVC).

Ⅵ Clinical Considerations of the Anterior Thorax *(Figure 2-1)*

A. **Insertion of a central venous catheter.** In clinical practice, access to the SVC and right side of heart is required to monitor blood pressure, long-term feeding, and administration of drugs. The internal jugular vein and subclavian vein are generally used.

1. **Internal jugular vein (central or anterior approach).** The needle is inserted at the apex of a triangle formed by the two heads of the sternocleidomastoid muscle and the clavicle of the right side.

2. **Subclavian vein (infraclavicular approach).** Place index finger at sternal notch and thumb at the intersection of the clavicle and first rib as anatomical landmarks. The needle is inserted below the clavicle and lateral to your thumb on the right side.

3. **Complications of a central venous catheter** may include: puncture of subclavian artery or subclavian vein, pneumothorax, hemothorax, trauma to trunks of brachial plexus, arrhythmias, venous thrombosis, erosion of catheter through the SVC, damage to tricuspid valve, and infections.

B. **Aortic aneurysm** may compress the trachea and tug on the trachea with each cardiac systole such that it can be felt by palpating the trachea at the sternal notch (T2).

C. **Aortic dissection** is a separation of the layers of the aortic wall initiated either by a tear in the weakened tunica intima or by a rupture of vasa vasorum with subintimal hemorrhage. Death from aortic dissection is usually from retrograde dissection of blood into pericardium (causing cardiac tamponade) or into the pleural space.

D. **Thoracic outlet syndrome** may be the result of an anomalous cervical rib and may compress the lower trunk of the brachial plexus and/or subclavian artery. Clinical findings include: atrophy of thenar and hypothenar eminences, atrophy of interosseous muscles, sensory deficits on medial side of forearm and hand, diminished radial artery pulse upon moving head to the opposite side, and a bruit over the subclavian artery.

E. **Aortic transection** is a result of a deceleration injury (e.g., high-speed motor vehicle accidents) in which the aorta tears just distal to the left subclavian artery. The tear is in a transverse direction and may involve all three tunics of the aorta.

F. **Knife wound to thorax above the clavicle** may damage the following structures at the root of the neck. The **subclavian artery** may be cut. The **lower trunk of the brachial plexus** may be cut causing loss of hand movements (ulnar nerve involvement) and loss of sensation over the medial aspect of the arm, forearm, and last two digits (C8 and T1 dermatomes). The **cervical pleura** and **apex of the lung** may be cut causing an open pneumothorax and collapse of the lung. These structures project superiorly into the neck through the thoracic inlet and posterior to the sternocleidomastoid muscle.

G. **Projections of the diaphragm on the thorax.** The **central tendon of the diaphragm** lies directly posterior to the xiphosternal joint. The **right dome** of the diaphragm arches superiorly to the **upper** border of rib 5 in the midclavicular line. The **left** dome of the diaphragm arches superiorly to the **lower** border of rib 5 in the midclavicular line.

H.   Scalene lymph node biopsy. Scalene lymph nodes are located behind the clavicle surrounded by pleura, lymph ducts, and the phrenic nerve. Inadvertent damage to the these structures causes the following clinical findings: pneumothorax, lymph leakage, and diaphragm paralysis, respectively.

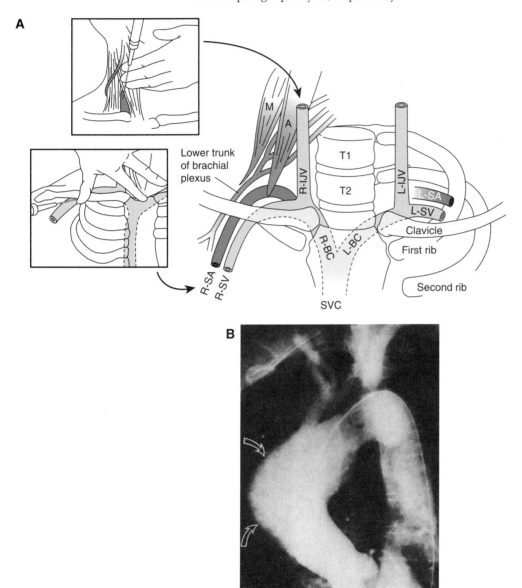

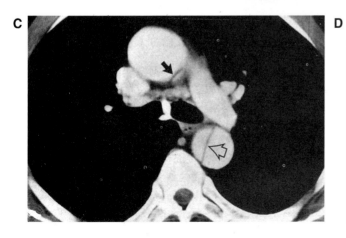

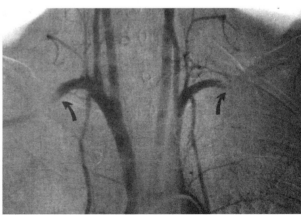

VII Clinical Considerations of the Lateral Thorax *(Figure 2-2A)*

A. **Intercostal nerve block.** An intercostal nerve block may be necessary to relieve pain associated with a rib fracture or herpes zoster (shingles). A needle is inserted at the posterior angle of the rib along the **lower** border of the rib to bathe the nerve in anesthetic. The needle penetrates the following structures: **skin → superficial fascia → serratus anterior muscle → external intercostal muscle → internal intercostal muscle.** Several intercostal nerves must be blocked to achieve pain relief because of the presence of nerve collaterals (i.e., overlapping of contiguous dermatomes).

B. **Tube thoracostomy.** Tube thoracostomy is performed to evacuate ongoing production of air/fluid into the pleural cavity. A tube is inserted through intercostal space 5 in the anterior axillary line (i.e., posterior approach) close to the **upper** border of the rib to avoid the **intercostal vein, artery,** and **nerve** that run in the costal groove between the internal intercostal muscle and innermost intercostal muscle. An incision is made at intercostal space 6 lateral to the nipple, but medial to the latissimus dorsi muscle. The tube will penetrate **skin → superficial fascia → serratus anterior muscle → external intercostal muscle → internal intercostal muscle → innermost intercostal muscle → parietal pleura.**

VIII Clinical Considerations of the Posterior Thorax *(Figure 2-2B)*

A. **Rib fractures.** The **middle ribs** are most commonly fractured just anterior to their **costal angle** (weakest point of the rib). A rib fracture on the right side may damage the **right kidney** and **liver.** A rib fracture on the left side may damage the **left kidney** and **spleen.** A rib fracture on either side may damage the **pleura** as it crosses rib 12. Rib fractures are generally associated with tearing of the intercostal muscles.

B. **Rib dislocation** refers to the displacement of the costal cartilage from the sternum.

C. **Rib separation** refers to a separation at the costochondral joint (i.e., between the rib and its costal cartilage).

IX Mediastinum *(Figure 2-2C)*

The mediastinum is the space between the pleural cavities in the thorax. It is bounded laterally by the pleural cavities, anteriorly by the sternum, and posteriorly by the vertebral column. The mediastinum is divided into the **superior, anterior, middle,** and **posterior** divisions.

A. **Superior mediastinum.** The contents of the superior mediastinum include: the trachea, esophagus, thymus, phrenic nerves, azygos vein, SVC, brachiocephalic artery and veins, aortic arch, left common carotid artery, left subclavian artery, and thoracic duct. Common pathologies found in this area include: **aortic arch aneurysm, esophageal perforation either from endoscopy or invading malignancy,** or **traumatic rupture of trachea.**

◄

FIGURE 2-1. (A) Anterior chest wall. The first pair of ribs are shown with their articulation with the T1 vertebra and manubrium of the sternum. On the right, structures crossing rib 1 are shown (subclavian vein, subclavian artery, and brachial plexus). Note the relationship of these structures to the clavicle. Note also the arrangement of the large veins in this area and their use in placing a central venous catheter (internal jugular vein [IJV] approach or subclavian approach). L-BC—left brachiocephalic vein; L-IJV—left internal jugular vein; L-SV—left subclavian vein; RBC—right brachiocephalic vein; R-IJV—right internal jugular vein; R-SA—right subclavian artery; R-SV—right subclavian vein; SVC—superior vena cava; **(B) Aortic aneurysm.** Angiogram shows an atherosclerotic aneurysm *(curved arrows)* protruding from the ascending aorta. **(C) Aortic dissection.** Computed tomography (CT) scan shows a tunica intima flap within the ascending *(closed arrow)* and descending *(open arrow)* aorta. The larger false lumen compresses the true lumen. **(D) Thoracic outlet syndrome.** Angiogram taken with abduction of both arms shows blood flow is partially occluded in the subclavian arteries *(arrows)*.

A

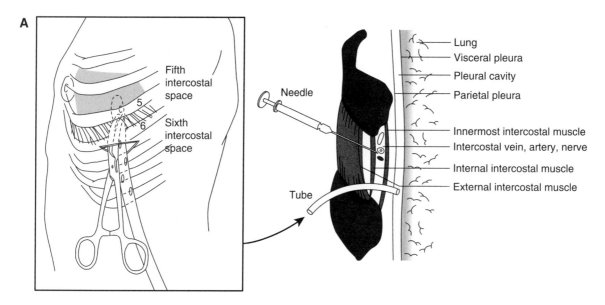

Fifth intercostal space

Sixth intercostal space

5

6

Needle

Tube

Lung

Visceral pleura

Pleural cavity

Parietal pleura

Innermost intercostal muscle

Intercostal vein, artery, nerve

Internal intercostal muscle

External intercostal muscle

B

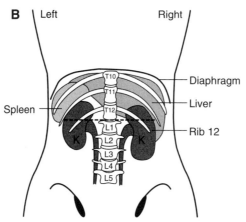

Left

Right

T10

T11

T12

L1

L2

L3

L4

L5

K

K

Spleen

Diaphragm

Liver

Rib 12

C

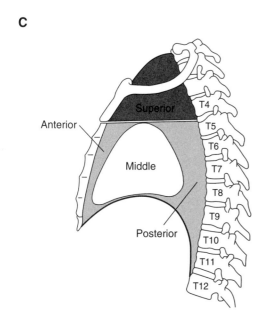

Anterior

Superior

Middle

Posterior

T4

T5

T6

T7

T8

T9

T10

T11

T12

D

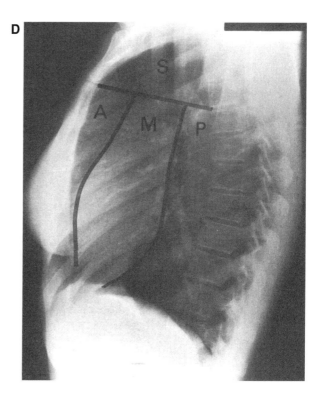

S

A

M

P

B. **Anterior mediastinum.** The contents of the anterior mediastinum include: the thymus, fat, lymph nodes, and connective tissue. Common pathologies found in this area include: **thymoma associated with myasthenia gravis and red blood cell (RBC) aplasia, thyroid mass, germinal cell neoplasm,** and **lymphomas (Hodgkin's or non-Hodgkin's).**

C. **Middle mediastinum.** The contents of the middle mediastinum include: the heart, pericardium, phrenic nerves, ascending aorta, SVC, inferior vena cava (IVC), and coronary arteries and veins. Common pathologies found in this area include: **pericardial cysts, bronchiogenic cysts,** and **sarcoidosis.**

D. **Posterior mediastinum.** The contents of the posterior mediastinum include: the descending aorta, esophagus, thoracic duct, azygos vein, splanchnic nerves, vagus nerves, and sympathetic trunk. Common pathologies found in this area include: **ganglioneuromas, neuroblastomas,** or **esophageal diverticula** or **neoplasms.**

THE HEART

The Pericardium

A. **General features.** The pericardium consists of three layers: the visceral layer of serous pericardium, the parietal layer of serous pericardium, and the fibrous pericardium.
 1. The **visceral layer of serous pericardium** (known histologically as the **epicardium**) consists of a layer of simple squamous epithelium (called **mesothelium**). Beneath the mesothelium, coronary arteries, coronary veins, and nerves travel along the surface of the heart in a thin collagen bed; adipose tissue is also present.
 2. The **parietal layer of serous pericardium.** At the base of the aorta and pulmonary trunk, the mesothelium of the visceral layer of serous pericardium is reflected and becomes continuous with the parietal layer of serous pericardium such that the parietal layer of serous pericardium also consists of a layer of **mesothelium.**
 3. The **pericardial cavity** lies between the visceral layer and parietal layer of serous pericardium and normally contains a small amount of pericardial fluid (20 mL), which allows friction-free movement of the heart during diastole and systole. The **transverse sinus** is a recess of the pericardial cavity. After the pericardial sac is opened, a surgeon can pass a finger or ligature (posterior to the aorta and pulmonary trunk and anterior to the SVC) from one side of the heart to the other through the transverse sinus. The **oblique sinus** is a recess of the pericardial cavity that ends in a cul-de-sac surrounded by the pulmonary veins.
 4. **Fibrous pericardium** is a thick (~1 mm) **collagen layer** (no elastic fibers) with **little ability to distend acutely.** The fibrous pericardium fuses superiorly to the tunica adventitia of the great vessels, inferiorly to the central tendon of the diaphragm, and anteriorly to the sternum. The **phrenic nerve** and **pericardio-**

◄
FIGURE 2-2. (A) Lateral chest wall. Diagram shows an intercostal space and layers. Note the location of the intercostal vein, artery, and nerve. Note the relationship of the intercostal space to the pleura and lung. Needle indicates the positioning for an intercostal nerve block. Tube indicates the positioning for a tube thoracostomy. The inset demonstrates the surgical approach to inserting a tube for tube thoracostomy. **(B) Posterior chest wall.** Note that the kidneys (*K*) are located from T12 to L3 vertebrae and that the right kidney is lower than the left. The pleura extends across rib 12 (*dotted line*). Note the structures that may be injured by fractures to the lower ribs. During a splenectomy, the left kidney may be damaged due to its close anatomical relationship and connection via the splenorenal ligament. **(C and D) Mediastinum. (C)** A diagram indicating the superior, anterior, middle, and posterior divisions of the mediastinum. **(D)** A lateral radiograph demarcates the superior (*S*), anterior (*A*), middle (*M*), and posterior (*P*) divisions of the mediastinum.

phrenic artery descend through the mediastinum lateral to the fibrous pericardium and are in jeopardy during surgery to the heart.

5. The **thoracic portion of the IVC** lies within the pericardium so the pericardium must be opened to expose this portion of the IVC.

B. Clinical considerations

1. **Cardiac tamponade (heart compression)** is the accumulation of fluid within the pericardial cavity, resulting in compression of the heart because the fibrous pericardium is inelastic. Clinical findings include: hypotension (blood pressure [BP] 90/40) that does not respond to rehydration, compression of the SVC that may cause the veins of the face and neck to engorge with blood, a distention of veins of the neck on inspiration (**Kussmaul sign**), paradoxical pulse (inspiratory lowering of BP by more than 10 mm Hg), the spontaneous filling of a syringe when blood is drawn due to increased venous pressure, and distant heart sounds.

2. **Pericardiocentesis** is the removal of fluid from the pericardial cavity, which can be approached in two ways.

   a. **Sternal approach.** A needle is inserted at intercostal space 5 or 6 on the left side near the sternum. The cardiac notch of the left lung leaves the fibrous pericardium exposed at this site. The needle penetrates the following structures: **skin → superficial fascia → pectoralis major muscle → external intercostal membrane → internal intercostal muscle → transverse thoracic muscle → fibrous pericardium → parietal layer of serous pericardium.** The internal thoracic artery, coronary arteries, and pleura may be damaged during this approach.

   b. **Subxiphoid approach.** A needle is inserted at the left infrasternal angle and is angled in a superior and posterior position. The needle penetrates the following structures: **skin → superficial fascia → anterior rectus sheath → rectus abdominus muscle → transverse abdominus muscle → fibrous pericardium → parietal layer of serous pericardium.** The diaphragm and liver may be damaged during this approach.

Ⅱ Heart Surfaces (Figure 2-3A and B)

The heart has six surfaces.

A. **Posterior surface (base)** consists mainly of the **left atrium,** which receives the pulmonary veins and is related to vertebral bodies T6-T9.

B. **Apex** consists of the inferior lateral portion of the **left ventricle** at intercostal space 5 along the midclavicular line. The maximal pulsation of the heart (apex beat) occurs at the apex.

C. **Anterior surface (sternocostal surface)** consists mainly of the **right ventricle.**

D. **Inferior surface (diaphragmatic surface)** consists mainly of the **left ventricle** and is related to the central tendon of the diaphragm.

E. **Left surface (pulmonary surface)** consists mainly of the left ventricle and occupies the cardiac impression of the left lung.

F. **Right surface** consists mainly of the right atrium located between the SVC and IVC.

Ⅲ Heart Borders (Figure 2-3A and B)

The heart has four borders.

A. **Right border** consists of the **right atrium, SVC, and IVC.**

B. **Left border** consists of the **left ventricle, left atrium, pulmonary trunk,** and **aortic arch.**

C. **Inferior border** consists of the **right ventricle.**

D. **Superior border** consists of the **right atrium, left atrium, SVC, ascending aorta,** and **pulmonary trunk.**

Fibrous Skeleton of the Heart *(Figure 2-3C)*

The fibrous skeleton is dense framework of collagen within the heart that: keeps the orifices of the atrioventricular valves and semilunar valve patent, provides an attachment site of the valve leaflets and cusps, serves as the origin and insertion sites of cardiac myocytes, and forms an electrical "barrier" between the atria and ventricles so that they contract independently. The fibrous skeleton consists of:

A. **Tricuspid annulus, mitral annulus, pulmonary annulus,** and **aortic annulus—four** fibrous rings (also called **annuli fibrosi**) that surround the orifices of the tricuspid valve, mitral valve, pulmonary semilunar valve, and aortic semilunar valve, respectively

B. **Right fibrous trigone** (largest and strongest component of the skeleton), **left fibrous trigone,** and **intervalvular trigone** formed by the collagen connecting all the fibrous rings

C. **Conus ligament (ligament of Krehl),** which is a small collagenous connection between the pulmonary and aortic valves

D. **Tendon of Todaro,** which extends from the tricuspid annulus

E. **Membranous septum,** which consists of an interventricular and atrioventricular portion

Valves and Auscultation Sites *(Figure 2-3D)*

A. **Tricuspid (right atrioventricular) valve.** The tricuspid valve is located between the right atrium and the right ventricle and is composed of **three leaflets (anterior, posterior,** and **septal leaflets),** all of which are tethered to **papillary muscles (anterior, posterior,** and **medial)** by **chorda tendineae.** The auscultation site is **over the sternum at intercostal space 5.**

B. **Bicuspid (mitral; left atrioventricular) valve.** The bicuspid valve is located between the left atrium and left ventricle and is composed of **two leaflets (anterior** and **posterior leaflets)** both of which are tethered to **papillary muscles (anterolateral** and **posteromedial)** by **chorda tendineae.** The auscultation site is at the **cardiac apex at left intercostal space 5.**

C. **Pulmonary semilunar valve (pulmonic valve).** The pulmonary semilunar valve is the outflow valve of the right ventricle and is composed of **three cusps (anterior, right,** and **left cusps)** that fit closely together when closed. The orifice of the pulmonary semilunar valve is directed to the left shoulder. The auscultation site is just **lateral to the sternum at left intercostal space 2.**

D. **Aortic semilunar valve.** The aortic semilunar valve is the outflow valve of the left ventricle and is composed of **three cusps (posterior, right,** and **left cusps)** that fit closely together when closed. The orifice of the aortic semilunar valve is directed to the right shoulder. The auscultation site is just **lateral to the sternum at right intercostal space 2.**

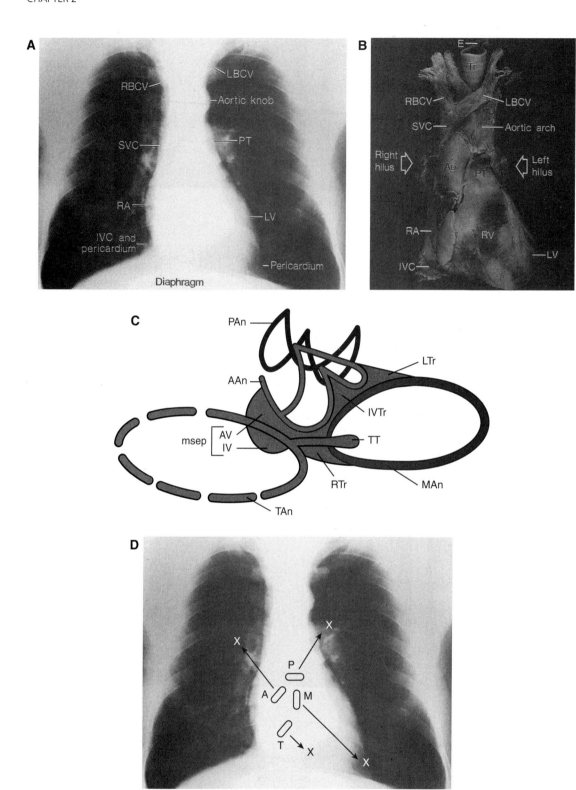

FIGURE 2-3. (A) Radiograph shows the various components of the heart and great vessels. **(B)** Photograph of the anatomical heart and great vessels for comparison to the radiograph in (A). Ao—aorta; E—esophagus; IVC—inferior vena cava; LBCV—left brachiocephalic vein; LV—left ventricle; PT—pulmonary trunk; RA—right atrium;. RBCV—right brachiocephalic vein; RV—right ventricle; SVC—superior vena cava; Tr—trachea. **(C) Diagram of the fibrous skeleton of the heart** (anterior view; same orientation as a CT or MRI scan). AAn—aortic annulus; IVTr—intervalvular trigone; LTr—left trigone; MAn—mitral annulus; MSep—membranous septum atrioventricular (AV) portion and interventricular (IV) portion; PAn—pulmonary annulus; RTr—right trigone; TAn—tricuspid annulus; TT—tendon of Todaro. **(D) Valve and auscultation sites.** The position of the heart valves are indicated on a radiograph. The locations where heart sounds are auscultated are indicated by an X. A—aortic valve; M—mitral valve; P—pulmonary valve; T—tricuspid valve. Arrows indicate the direction of blood flow.

E. **Heart sounds**
1. S_1 **(first sound; "lub" sound)** is caused by closure of the tricuspid and bicuspid valves.
2. S_2 **(second sound; "dub" sound)** is cause by closure of the pulmonary and aortic valves.

VI Vasculature of the Heart (*Figure 2-4*)

A. **Arterial supply.** The right coronary artery (RCA) and left coronary artery supply oxygenated arterial blood to the heart. The coronary arteries fill with blood during diastole. The coronary arteries have maximal blood flow during diastole and minimal blood flow during systole.
1. **Right coronary artery.** The RCA arises from the right aortic sinus (of Valsalva) of the ascending aorta and courses in the coronary sulcus. The blood supply of the heart is considered **right-side dominant** (most common) if the posterior interventricular artery arises from the RCA. The RCA branches into: the **sinoatrial (SA) nodal artery, conus branch, right marginal artery, atrioventricular (AV) nodal artery, terminal branches, posterior interventricular artery,** and **septal branches.**
2. **Left main coronary artery (LMCA).** The LMCA arises from the left aortic sinus (of Valsalva) of the ascending aorta. The blood supply of the heart is considered **left-side dominant** (less common) if the posterior interventricular artery arises from the LMCA. The LMCA branches into the:
    a. **Left circumflex artery (LCx),** which further branches into: the **anterior marginal artery, obtuse marginal artery, atrial branches,** and **posterior marginal artery**
    b. **Intermediate ramus** (a variable branch)
    c. **Anterior interventricular artery** (also called left anterior descending artery [LAD]), which further branches into: the anterior diagonal artery and septal branches

B. **Venous drainage**
1. **Coronary sinus** is the largest vein draining the heart and drains directly into the right atrium. At the opening of the coronary sinus, a crescent-shaped valve remnant (the **thebesian valve**) is present.
2. **Great cardiac vein** follows the **anterior interventricular artery** and drains into the coronary sinus.
3. **Middle cardiac vein** follows the **posterior interventricular artery** and drains into the coronary sinus.
4. **Small cardiac vein** follows the **right marginal artery** and drains into the coronary sinus.
5. **Oblique vein of the left atrium** is a remnant of the embryonic left SVC and drains into the coronary sinus.
6. **Left posterior ventricular vein** drains into the coronary sinus.
7. **Left marginal vein** drains into the coronary sinus.
8. **Anterior cardiac veins** are found on the anterior aspect of the right ventricle and drain directly into the right atrium.
9. **Smallest cardiac veins** begin within the wall of the heart and drain directly into the nearest heart chamber.

VII The Conduction System (*Figure 2-5A*)

A. **Sinoatrial node** is the **pacemaker** of the heart and is located at the junction of the SVC and right atrium just beneath the epicardium. From the SA node, the impulse spreads throughout the right atrium and to the AV node via the **anterior, middle, posterior**

Arterial Supply

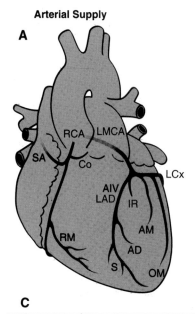

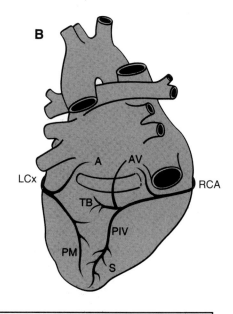

C

	Branches	Structures Supplied
Right coronary artery	SA nodal artery Conus branch Right marginal artery AV nodal artery Terminal branches Posterior interventricular artery Septal branches	SA node Right atrium Right ventricle Diaphragmatic surface of the left ventricle AV node Posterior third of the interventricular septum

Left main coronary artery	**Left circumflex artery**
	    Anterior marginal artery
	    Obtuse marginal artery
	    Atrial branches
	    Posterior marginal artery
	Intermediate ramus
	Anterior interventricular artery (left anterior descending)
	    Anterior diagonal artery
	    Septal branches
		Left atrium
		Majority of the left ventricle
		Right and left bundle branches of the bundle of His
		Anterior two-thirds of the interventricular septum

Venous Drainage

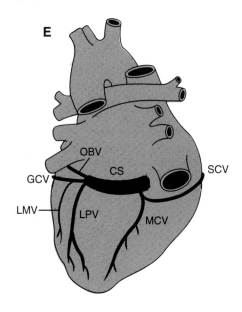

and **internodal tracts** and to the left atrium via the **Bachmann bundle.** If all SA node activity is destroyed, the AV node assumes the pacemaker role.

B. **Atrioventricular node** is located on the right side of the AV portion of the atrial septum near the ostium of the coronary sinus in the subendocardial space. The AV septum corresponds to the **triangle of Koch,** an important anatomical landmark because it contains the AV node and the proximal penetrated portion of the bundle of His.

C. **Bundle of His, bundle branches, Purkinje myocytes.** The **bundle of His** travels in the subendocardial space on the right side of the interventricular septum and divides into the **right and left bundle branches.** The left bundle branch is thicker than the right bundle branch. A portion of the right bundle branch enters the septomarginal trabeculae (moderator band) to supply the anterior papillary muscle. The left bundle branch further divides into an **anterior segment** and **posterior segment.** The right and left bundle branches both terminate in a complex network of intramural **Purkinje myocytes.**

Ⅷ Innervation of the Heart *(Figure 2-5B)*

The heart is innervated by the **superficial cardiac plexus,** which is located inferior to the aortic arch and anterior to the right pulmonary artery, and by the **deep cardiac plexus,** which is located posterior to the aortic arch and anterior to the tracheal bifurcation. These plexuses contain **both parasympathetic (vagus; cranial nerve [CN] X) and sympathetic components.**

A. **Parasympathetic.** Preganglionic neuronal cell bodies are located in the **dorsal nucleus of the vagus** and **nucleus ambiguus** of the medulla. Preganglionic axons run in the **vagus (CN X) nerve.** Postganglionic neuronal cell bodies are located in the cardiac plexus and atrial wall. Postganglionic axons are distributed to the **SA node, AV node, atrial myocytes (not ventricular myocytes),** and **smooth muscle of coronary arteries,** causing a **decrease in heart rate,** a **decrease in conduction velocity through the AV node,** and a **decrease in contractility of atrial myocytes.** Postganglionic axons release **acetylcholine (ACh)** as a neurotransmitter. ACh binds to the **M$_2$ muscarinic ACh receptor (mAChR),** which is a G-protein–linked receptor that inhibits adenylate cyclase and decreases cyclic adenosine monophosphate (cAMP) levels. The SA node and AV node contain high levels of **acetylcholinesterase** (degrades ACh rapidly) such that any given vagal stimulation is **short-lived. Vasovagal syncope** is a brief period of lightheadedness or loss of consciousness due to an intense burst of CN X activity. Afferent (sensory) neurons of CN X whose cell bodies are located in the nodose ganglion innervate **baroreceptors** in the great veins, atria, and aortic arch and relay **changes in blood pressure** to the solitary nucleus within the central nervous system (CNS). Afferent (sensory) neurons of CN X whose cell bodies are located in the nodose ganglion innervate **chemoreceptors** (specifically the **aortic bodies**) and relay **changes in partial arterial pressure of oxygen (Pao$_2$)** to the solitary nucleus within the CNS.

B. **Sympathetic.** Preganglionic neuronal cell bodies are located in the **intermediolateral columns** of the spinal cord. Preganglionic axons enter the paravertebral ganglion and travel to the stellate/middle cervical ganglia. Postganglionic neuronal cell bodies are

◀

FIGURE 2-4. (A and B) Arterial supply of the heart. (A) Anterior (sternocostal) surface of the heart. (B) Inferior (diaphragmatic) surface of the heart. A—atrial branches; AD—anterior diagonal artery; AIV—anterior interventricular artery; AV—atrioventricular nodal artery; Co—conus branch; IR—intermediate ramus; LAD—left anterior descending artery; LCx—left circumflex artery; LMCA—left main coronary artery; OM—obtuse marginal artery; PIV—posterior interventricular artery; PM—posterior marginal artery; RCA—right coronary artery; RM—right marginal artery; S—septal branches; SA—sinoatrial nodal artery; TB—terminal branches. **(C)** Table indicates the branches of the right and left coronary arteries and the structures supplied by each. **(D and E) Venous drainage of the heart. (D) Anterior (sternocostal) surface of the heart. (E) Inferior (diaphragmatic) surface of the heart.** ACV—anterior cardiac veins; CS—coronary sinus; GCV—great cardiac vein; LMV—left marginal vein; LPV—left posterior vein; MCV—middle cardiac vein; OBV—oblique vein of the left atrium; SCV—small cardiac vein.

A

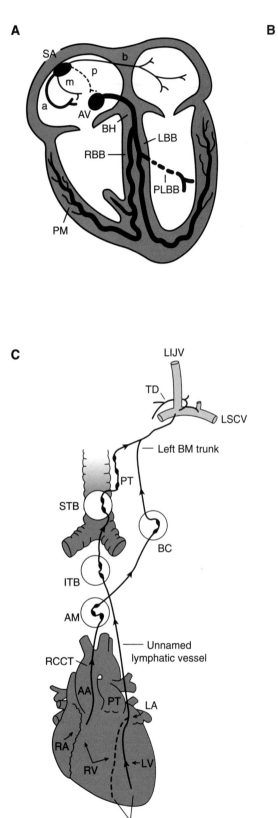

B

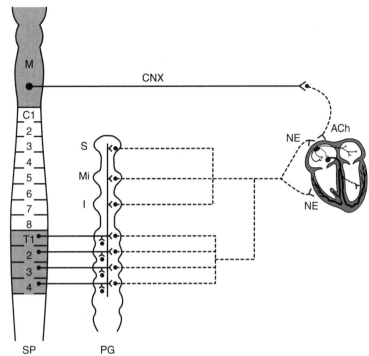

C

located in the **stellate** and **middle cervical ganglia.** Postganglionic axons are distributed to the **SA node, AV node, atrial myocytes, ventricular myocytes,** and **smooth muscle of coronary arteries** causing an **increase in heart rate,** an **increase in conduction velocity through the AV node,** and an **increase in contractility of atrial and ventricular myocytes.** Postganglionic axons release **norepinephrine (NE)** as a neurotransmitter. NE binds to the β_1-**adrenergic receptor,** which is a G-protein–linked receptor that stimulates adenylate cyclase and increases cAMP levels. Released NE is either carried away by the bloodstream or taken up by the nerve terminals so that sympathetic stimulation is relatively **long-lived.** Afferent (sensory) neurons whose cell bodies are located in the dorsal root ganglion run with the sympathetic nerves and relay **pain** information to T1-T5 spinal cord segments within the CNS. The pain associated with angina pectoris or a "heart attack" may be referred over the T1-T5 dermatomes (i.e., the classic referred pain down the left arm).

Ⓘ Lymphatic Drainage of the Heart *(Figure 2-5C)*

The adult heart has lymphatic plexuses that communicate freely within the substance of the heart called: the **subendocardial plexus, myocardial plexus,** and **subepicardial plexus.** The subendocardial and myocardial plexuses drain into the subepicardial plexus, which coalesces into the **right cardiac collecting trunk** and **left cardiac collecting trunk.** The right and left cardiac collecting trunks predominantly drain into the **left bronchomediastinal trunk,** which empties into the junction of the left internal jugular vein and left subclavian vein.

A. **Right cardiac collecting trunk** drains the right atrium and part of the right ventricle (right border and inferior surface), travels in the coronary sulcus near the right coronary artery, and ascends anterior to the ascending aorta to empty into the **anterior mediastinal nodes → left brachiocephalic nodes (most commonly) → left bronchomediastinal trunk.**

B. **Left cardiac collecting trunk** drains the left atrium, part of the right ventricle, and the left ventricle. One branch of the left cardiac collecting trunk travels in the anterior interventricular sulcus. Another branch of the left cardiac collecting trunk travels in the posterior interventricular sulcus. The two branches join in the coronary sulcus to form a large unnamed lymphatic vessel. The unnamed lymphatic vessel ascends between the pulmonary trunk and left atrium to empty into the **inferior tracheobronchial nodes → superior tracheobronchial nodes → paratracheal nodes → left bronchomediastinal trunk.**

Ⓧ Gross Anatomy Structure Overview *(Figure 2-6)*

A. **Right atrium.** The right atrium receives venous blood from the SVC, IVC, and coronary sinus. The right atrium consists of: the **right auricle,** which is a conical, muscular pouch; **pectinate muscles** that form the trabeculated part of the right atrium (2–4 mm thick) and develop embryologically from the primitive atrium; the **sinus venarum,** which is the smooth part of the right atrium and develops embryologically from the sinus venous; the **crista terminalis** (an internal muscular ridge 3–6 mm thick), which

◀

FIGURE 2-5. (A) Diagram of the conduction system of the heart. a—anterior internodal tract; AV—atrioventricular node; b—Bachmann bundle; BH—bundle of His; LBB—left bundle branch; m—middle internodal tract; p—posterior internodal tract;. pLBB—posterior segment of the left bundle branch; PM—Purkinje myocytes; RBB—right bundle branch; SA—sinoatrial node. **(B) Innervation of the heart.** Parasympathetic innervation involving the vagus nerve (CN X) is shown. Sympathetic innervation is also shown. All preganglionic neurons are indicated by solid lines. All postganglionic neurons are indicated by dotted lines. ACh—acetylcholine; I—inferior cervical ganglion; M—medulla; Mi—middle cervical ganglion; PG—paravertebral ganglia; NE—norepinephrine; S—superior cervical ganglion; SP—spinal cord. **(C) Lymphatic drainage of the heart.** Diagram indicates the pattern of the right cardiac collecting trunk (*RCCT*) and left cardiac collecting trunk (*LCCT*). The arrows indicate the direction of lymph drainage from the right atrium (*RA*), right ventricle (*RV*), left ventricle (*LV*), and left atrium (*LA*). AA—ascending aorta; AM—anterior mediastinal nodes; BC—brachiocephalic nodes; BM—bronchomediastinal; ITB—inferior tracheobronchial nodes; LIJV—left internal jugular vein; LSCV—left subclavian vein; PT—paratracheal nodes; PT—pulmonary trunk; STB—superior tracheobronchial nodes; TD—thoracic duct.

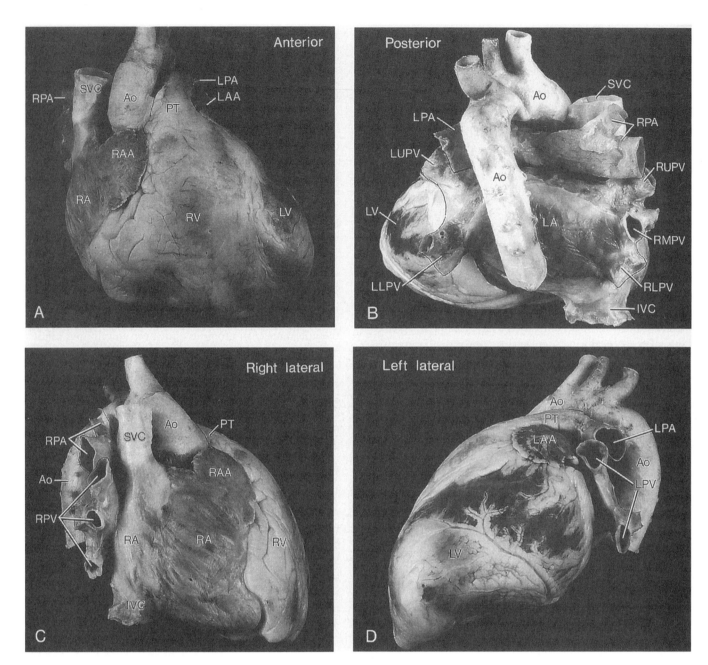

FIGURE 2-6. External heart anatomy. (A) Anterior view. **(B)** Posterior view. **(C)** Right lateral view. **(D)** Left lateral view.

(continued)

marks the junction between the trabeculated part and the smooth part of the right atrium; the **sulcus terminalis** (an external shallow groove), which also marks the junction between the trabeculated part and smooth part of the right atrium; the **openings of the SVC, IVC, coronary sinus, and the anterior cardiac vein; atrial septum,** which consists of an interatrial portion and AV portion; the **fossa ovalis,** which is an oval depression on the interatrial portion consisting of the **valve of the fossa ovalis** (a central sheet of thin fibrous tissue), a remnant of septum primum; and the **limbus of the fossa ovalis** (a horseshoe-shaped muscular rim), which is a remnant of the septum secundum. The wall of the right atrium between the pectinate muscles is < 1 mm thick and can be easily perforated by a catheter or pacemaker lead.

   B. **Right ventricle.** The trabeculated inflow tract of the right ventricle receives venous blood from the right atrium posteriorly through the tricuspid valve, whereas the

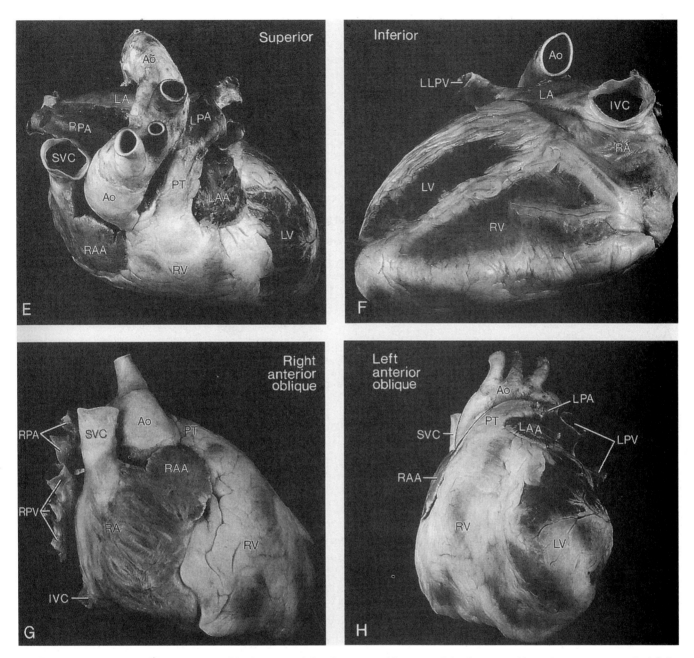

FIGURE 2-6. *(continued)* **(E)** Superior view. **(F)** Inferior view. **(G)** Right anterior oblique view. **(H)** Left anterior oblique view. Ao—aorta; IVC—inferior vena cava; LAA—left atrial appendage; LLPV—left lower pulmonary vein; LPA—left pulmonary artery; LUPV—left upper pulmonary vein; LV—left ventricle; PT—pulmonary trunk; RA—right atrium; RAA—right atrial appendage; RLPV—right lower pulmonary vein; RMPV—right middle pulmonary vein; RPA—right pulmonary artery; RPV—right pulmonary vein; RUPV—right upper pulmonary vein; RV—right ventricle; SVC—superior vena cava.

smooth outflow tract of the right ventricle expels blood superiorly and to the left into the pulmonary trunk. The right ventricle consists of: the **trabeculae carneae** (irregular muscular ridges), which form the trabeculated part of the right ventricle (inflow tract) and develop embryologically from the primitive ventricle; the **conus arteriosus (infundibulum),** which is the smooth part of the right ventricle (outflow tract) and develops embryologically from the bulbus cordis; the **supraventricular crest** (a C-shaped internal muscular ridge), which marks the junction between the trabeculated part and smooth part of the right ventricle; the **tricuspid valve (anterior, posterior, and septal cusps),** which attach at their base to the fibrous skeleton; the **chordae tendineae,** which are cords that extend from the free edge of the tricuspid valve to the papillary muscles and prevent eversion of the tricuspid valve into the right atrium, thereby preventing regurgitation of ventricular blood into the right atrium during systole; the **papillary muscles (anterior, posterior, and septal)**, which are conical muscular projections from the ventricular wall and are attached to the chordae tendineae; **interventricular (IV) septum**, which consists of a **membranous part** (located in a superior posterior position and continuous with the fibrous skeleton) and a **muscular part; septomarginal trabeculae (moderator band)**, which is a curved muscular bundle that extends from the IV septum to the anterior papillary muscle and contains part of the right bundle branch of the bundle of His to the anterior papillary muscle; **right AV orifice; opening of the pulmonary trunk; pulmonary semilunar valve (anterior, right, and left cusps)**, which lies at the apex of the conus arteriosus and prevents blood from returning to the right ventricle. In fetal and neonatal life, the thickness of the right ventricular wall is similar to the thickness of the left ventricular wall because of the equalization of pulmonary and aortic pressures by the ductus arteriosus. By 3 months of age, the infant heart shows regression of the right ventricular wall thickness.

C. **Left atrium.** The left atrium receives oxygenated blood from the lungs through the pulmonary veins. The left atrium consists of: the **left auricle,** which is a tubular muscular pouch; **pectinate muscles,** which form the trabeculated part of the left atrium and develop embryologically from the primitive atrium; the **smooth part of the left atrium,** which develops embryologically by incorporation of the transient common pulmonary vein into its wall; **openings of the valveless pulmonary veins; atrial septum,** which consists only of an interatrial portion; and **semilunar depression,** which indicates the valve of the fossa ovalis. The limbus of the fossa ovalis and the AV septum are not visible from the left atrium.

D. **Left ventricle.** The trabeculate inflow tract of the left ventricle receives oxygenated blood from the left atrium through the mitral valve, whereas the smooth outflow tract of the left ventricle expels blood superoanteriorly into the ascending aorta. The left ventricle consists of: the **trabeculae carneae** (irregular muscular ridges), which form the trabeculated part of the left ventricle (inflow tract) and develop embryologically from the primitive ventricle; **aortic vestibule,** which is the smooth part of the left ventricle (outflow tract) and develops embryologically from the bulbus cordis; **mitral valve (anterior** and **posterior cusps),** which attach at their base to the fibrous skeleton; **chordae tendineae,** which are cords that extend from the free edge of the mitral valve to the papillary muscles and prevent eversion of the mitral valve into the left atrium, thereby preventing regurgitation of ventricular blood into the left atrium during systole; **papillary muscles (anterior** and **posterior),** which are conical muscular projections from the ventricular wall and are attached to the chordae tendineae; **left AV orifice; opening of the ascending aorta; aortic semilunar valve (posterior, right, and left cusps),** which lies at the apex of the aortic vestibule and prevents blood from returning to the left ventricle.

Chapter 3

Radiology

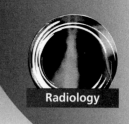

❶ Radiographs

A. **Posteroanterior (PA) chest film.** The film cassette is placed against the chest, and the x-ray beam is directed at the back and travels in a posterior-anterior direction (hence the name). The routine PA chest film is taken with the patient upright and in full inspiration. A normal chest film shows four densities listed from less radiodense (black) → more radiodense (white): the air density of the lungs; fat density around the muscles; water density of the heart, muscle, and blood; and bone density of the ribs and vertebrae.

B. **Anteroposterior (AP) chest film.** The film cassette is placed against the back, and the x-ray beam is directed at the chest and travels in an anterior-posterior direction. The AP chest film is usually performed on very sick patients who are unable to stand and on infants. The patient is usually supine or sitting in bed.

C. **Lateral chest film.** The film cassette is placed against the left side of the chest, and the x-ray is directed at the right side of the chest and travels from the right side to the left side.

D. **Oblique chest film.** The right anterior oblique and left anterior oblique views represent intermediary positions between the PA and lateral views.

E. **Radiology highlights**
1. There are **six causes of left atrium enlargement:** aortic valve stenosis or insufficiency, mitral valve stenosis or insufficiency, intracardiac shunts (e.g., ventricular septal defect [VSD] or patent ductus arteriosus [PDA]), left ventricular failure, cardiac restriction, and diastolic dysfunction (e.g., old age, hypertension).
2. There are **five causes of left ventricle enlargement:** aortic valve insufficiency, end-stage mitral valve regurgitation, intracardiac shunts, left-sided heart failure, and end-stage hypertension.
3. There are **eight causes of right ventricle enlargement:** pulmonary embolus, pulmonary hypertension, pulmonic stenosis, pulmonic valve insufficiency, atrial septal defect (ASD), VSD, tricuspid regurgitation, and congenital disorders.
4. There are **five causes of right atrium enlargement:** right ventricular failure, tricuspid valve insufficiency, pulmonic stenosis, intracardiac shunts (e.g., ASD, VSD), and congenital disorders (e.g., Ebstein anomaly). Right atrium enlargement is difficult to assess radiographically. In most cases of right atrium enlargement, the right ventricle is also enlarged so that determination of the size of the right atrium is difficult. Isolated right atrium enlargement is uncommon.

❷ Angiography

Coronary angiography is the clinical gold standard for the diagnosis of coronary artery disease. A stenosis of > 50% constitutes significant coronary artery disease. There are three major views used in angiography, as indicated below.

A. **Right anterior oblique (RAO) view** with different cranial and caudal angulations

B. Left anterior oblique (LAO) view with different cranial and caudal angulations

C. Anteroposterior (AP) view with different cranial and caudal angulations

D. Angiography highlights
1. **The angiographic characteristics of a normal coronary artery** include: well opacified, runs its course without any interruptions or local decreases in diameter, and tapers off gradually.
2. **Coronary artery stenosis** is described in the following ways: its position along the course of the coronary artery (i.e., ostial, proximal, mid, distal, or at the bifurcation); native versus in-stent; focal or diffuse; concentric or eccentric; clear or hazy borders; presence or absence of calcification; presence or absence of a thrombus.
3. **The angiographic characteristics of the right coronary artery (RCA)** include: the right main coronary artery (RMCA) arises from the right aortic sinus (of Valsalva) at a point slightly inferior to the ostium of the left main coronary artery (LMCA), travels in the right atrioventricular (AV) groove toward the crux, and is divided into a proximal horizontal portion, a mid horizontal portion, and a distal vertical portion.
4. The **proximal and mid horizontal portions of the RCA** are visualized optimally in the LAO view. The **distal vertical portion of the RCA** is visualized optimally in the RAO view.
5. **The angiographic characteristics of the LMCA** include: the LMCA arises from the left aortic sinus (of Valsalva), travels posterior to the right ventricle outflow tract, extends for < 10 mm, and has a diameter of 4–6 mm.
6. The **ostium of the LMCA** is visualized optimally in the AP view. The **main course of the LMCA** is visualized optimally in the RAO view. The **bifurcation of the LMCA** into the left anterior descending artery (LAD) and left circumflex artery (LCx) is visualized optimally in the LAO caudal view (spider view).
7. The most common coronary artery anomaly is the absence of the LMCA, whereby the LAD and the LCx arise from separate aortic ostia. This is of practical clinical significance in that when contrast material is injected into the ostium of the LAD, one might mistakenly diagnose an occluded LCx.
8. The second most common coronary artery anomaly is the origin of the LCx from the RCA or from the right aortic sinus (of Valsalva).

Ⓘⓘ Echocardiography

Echocardiography (cardiac ultrasound) is the most powerful diagnostic tool for cardiac imaging and hemodynamics. There are a number of echocardiographic techniques, which include the following:

A. Motion-mode (M-mode) echocardiography displays the motion of the heart in a one-dimensional recording over time on a cathode ray tube or a paper strip tracing. M-mode echocardiography by itself is rarely used today. Clinical applications include: measurements of cardiac wall thickness and chamber diameter and temporal resolution of cardiac valve motion.

B. Doppler echocardiography (DE) displays the direction, turbulence, and velocity of blood flow to evaluate interruptions or obstructions in cardiac blood flow. DE is most useful in assessing cardiac valve disease, which results in characteristically altered cardiac blood flow. Clinical applications include: measurements of stroke volume, right ventricle output, systolic and diastolic ventricular function, intracardiac shunts, regurgitation flows, and cardiac valve function (most valuable use).

C. **Stress echocardiography** displays images of stress-induced cardiac wall abnormalities to evaluate myocardial ischemia in pre-stress and post-stress conditions. Clinical applications include: measurements of ejection fraction, ventricular function, regional cardiac wall motion, myocardial thickening, and cardiac function at baseline, as well as at maximal stress or point of symptoms; assessment of mitral valve stenosis, hypertrophic cardiomyopathy, coarctation of the aorta, and dysfunctional prosthetic valves; and, diagnosis of ischemic heart disease (most common use).

D. **Transesophageal echocardiography (TEE)** displays high-resolution cardiac images from the esophageal or gastric window rather than the chest wall. TEE combines cardiac ultrasound and upper gastrointestinal endoscopy. TEE allows high resolution of posterior heart structures (e.g., atria, interatrial septum, aorta) and circumvents acoustic shadowing due to ultrasound reflectors (e.g., prosthetic valves). Clinical applications include: assessment of native or prosthetic valve disease, infectious endocarditis, aortic or atrial abnormalities, and aortic dissection; evaluation of trauma victims; determination of the source of emboli in unexplained cerebral ischemia patients; and intraoperative monitoring during cardiac valve or high-risk surgery.

E. **2-D Echocardiography (cross-sectional)** displays real-time, tomographic images of the heart. Clinical applications include: depiction of anatomical relationships, cardiac wall motion, cardiac valve motion, intracardiac shunts, intracardiac masses (e.g., vegetations, thrombi, tumors), and movement of cardiac structures relative to one another. There are four major echocardiographic windows: **parasternal window** (long-axis and short-axis), **apical window, subcostal window** (coronal and sagittal), and **suprasternal window** (long-axis and short-axis). There are four major views in 2-D echocardiography that are used clinically:
    1. **Parasternal long-axis view,** which shows the right ventricle, right ventricle free wall, left ventricle, left ventricle posterior wall, left atrium, interventricular septum, aorta, aortic semilunar valve, mitral valve, posterior papillary muscle, and the anterior and posterior portions of the pericardial space
    2. **Parasternal short-axis view,** which shows the right ventricle, left ventricle, and mitral valve
    3. **Apical four-chamber view,** which shows the right ventricle, right ventricle free wall, left ventricle, left ventricle lateral wall, apex, right atrium, left atrium, interventricular septum, tricuspid valve, and mitral valve
    4. **Apical two-chamber view,** which shows the left ventricle, left ventricle inferior wall, left ventricle anterior wall, mitral valve, and left atrium

Ⅳ Radiographs, Magnetic Resonance Images, Angiograms, and Echocardiograms

A. **Normal cardiac series of radiographs** *(Figure 3-1)*

B. **Radiographs of normal, left atrium enlargement, left ventricle enlargement, and right ventricle enlargement** *(Figure 3-2)*

C. **Angiograms of the right and left main coronary arteries** *(Figure 3-3)*

D. **Diagram of 2-D transthoracic echocardiograms windows and standard 2-D echocardiograms** *(Figure 3-4)*

E. **Magnetic resonance images at six different levels** *(Figure 3-5)*

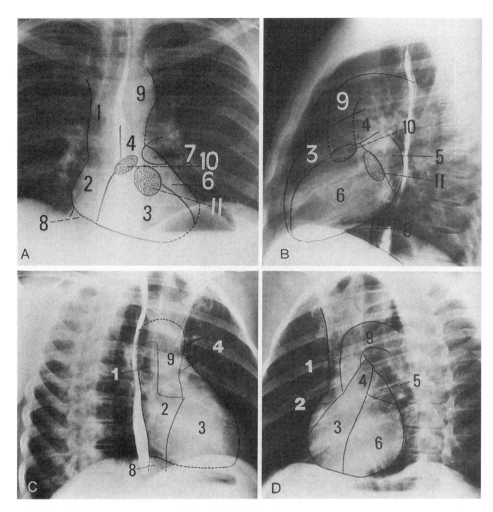

1: Superior vena cava
2: Right atrium
3: Right ventricle
4: Pulmonary outflow tract
5: Left atrium
6: Left ventricle
7: Left atrial appendage
8: Inferior vena cava
9: Ascending aorta and aortic arch
10: Aortic valve
11: Mitral valve

FIGURE 3-1. Normal cardiac series. (A) PA view. **(B)** Lateral view. **(C)** Right anterior oblique. **(D)** Left anterior oblique.

▶

FIGURE 3-2. (A–C) Normal heart. (A) PA radiograph shows the important structures on the left and right side of the heart. Note that the normal left atrial appendage is concave in appearance, not convex. **(B)** Lateral radiograph shows the important structures seen in this view of the heart. Note that on a lateral view the right heart is anterior and the left heart is posterior. **(C)** PA radiograph shows the normal measurements of heart width (~ 12 cm) and thorax width (~ 28 cm). This gives a cardiothoracic ratio of 0.43. The upper limit of normal is 0.5. for an individual patient, an increase in 1 cm in heart width from a prior radiograph is a very reliable index of heart enlargement. **(D and E) Left atrium enlargement. (D)** PA radiograph shows the upper left heart border enlarged in a lateral direction and the left atrial appendage convex, which is the most sensitive radiographic sign of elevated left atrium pressure or volume. A "double density" may also be observed just inferior to the carina. **(E)** Lateral radiograph shows the upper left heart border enlarged in a posterior direction (*arrow*). **(F and G) Left ventricle enlargement. (F)** PA radiograph shows the lower left heart border enlarged in a lateral direction (*arrow*) and the cardiac apex enlarged in an inferior and lateral direction. In left ventricle enlargement, the aorta is prominent and the pulmonary arteries are normal. **(G)** Lateral radiograph shows the lower left heart border enlarged in an inferior and posterior direction (*arrow*). **(H and I) Right ventricle enlargement. (H)** PA radiograph shows the right heart border enlarged in a lateral direction (*arrow*). In right ventricle enlargement, the aorta is diminutive and the pulmonary arteries are often prominent. **(I)** Lateral radiograph shows the right heart border enlarged in a superior and anterior direction (*arrow*). The normal right heart contacts the lower third of the sternum, whereas an enlarged right heart contacts the lower half of the sternum.

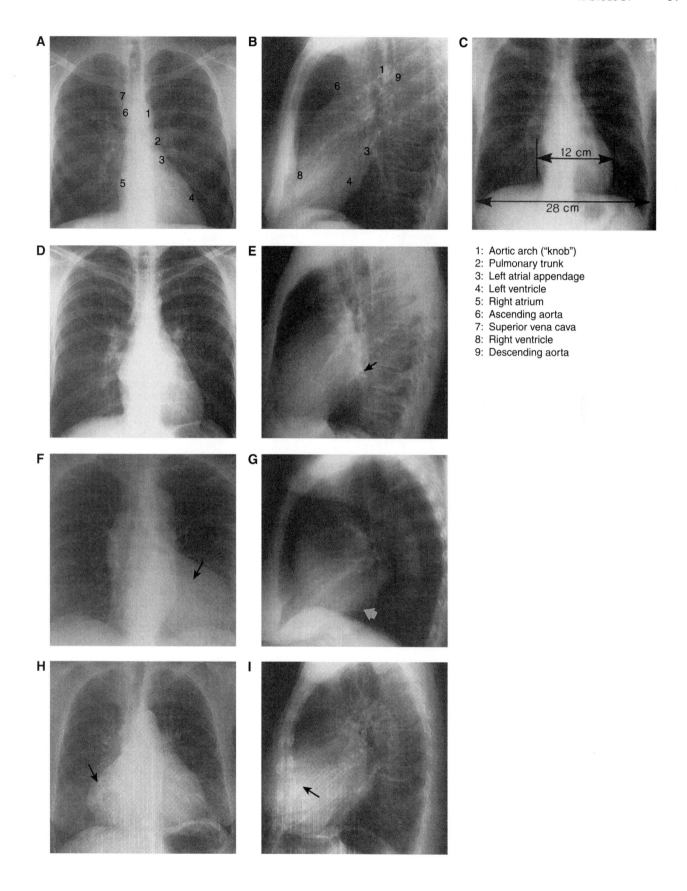

1: Aortic arch ("knob")
2: Pulmonary trunk
3: Left atrial appendage
4: Left ventricle
5: Right atrium
6: Ascending aorta
7: Superior vena cava
8: Right ventricle
9: Descending aorta

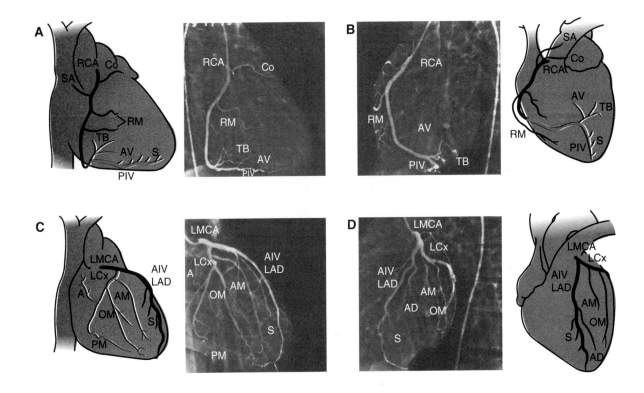

FIGURE 3-3. Angiograms of the right and left main coronary arteries. (A and B) Right coronary artery (RCA). (A) Right anterior oblique (RAO) angiogram shows the various branches of the RCA that can be observed in this view. **(B)** Left anterior oblique (LAO) angiogram shows the various branches of the RCA that can be observed in this view. **(C and D) Left main coronary artery (LMCA). (C)** Right anterior oblique angiogram shows the various branches of the LMCA that can be observed in this view. **(D)** Left anterior oblique (LAO) angiogram shows the various branches of the LMCA that can be observed in this view. A—atrial branches; AD—anterior diagonal artery; AIV—anterior interventricular artery; AV—atrioventricular nodal artery; Co—conus branch; LAD—left anterior descending artery; LCx—left circumflex artery; OM—obtuse marginal artery; PIV—posterior interventricular artery, PM—posterior marginal artery; RCA—right coronary artery; RM—right marginal artery; S—septal branches; SA—sinoatrial nodal artery; TB—terminal branches.

FIGURE 3-4. Diagram of 2-D transthoracic echocardiographic windows. (A and B) Parasternal window. (A) Parasternal long axis. The anatomy of the various planes (1, 2, and 3) is shown. Note that the view through plane 2 is one of the standard echocardiograms routinely used in clinical practice and is commonly called the **parasternal long-axis view(*). (B) Parasternal short axis.** The anatomy of the various planes (1, 2, and 3) is shown. Note that the view through plane 2 is one of the standard echocardiograms routinely used in clinical practice and is commonly called the **parasternal short-axis view (*). (C) Apical window.** The anatomy of the various planes (1, 2, and 3) is shown. Note that the view through plane 1 is commonly called the **5-chamber view** (i.e., right atrium, right ventricle, left atrium, left ventricle, and ascending aorta). Note that the view through plane 2 is one of the standard echocardiograms routinely used in clinical practice and is commonly called the **4-chamber view (*).** Note that if the transducer is angled slightly during the 4-chamber view, a **3-chamber view** can be obtained (i.e., left atrium, left ventricle, and ascending aorta), which is similar in appearance to the parasternal long axis view (plane 2) such that this view is sometimes called the **apical long-axis view.** Note that if the transducer is angled perpendicularly during the 4-chamber view, a **2-chamber view** can be obtained (i.e., left atrium, and left ventricle), which is one of the standard echocardiograms routinely used in clinical practice **(*). (D and E) Subcostal window. (D) Subcostal coronal axis.** The anatomy of the various planes (1, 2, 3, and 4) is shown. **(E) Subcostal sagittal axis.** The anatomy of the various planes (1, 2, 3, and 4) is shown. **(F and G) Suprasternal window. (F) Suprasternal long axis.** The anatomy of planes 1 and 2 is shown. **(G) Suprasternal short axis.** The anatomy of planes 1 and 2 is shown. Ao—aorta; AP—apex; av—aortic semilunar valve; CS—coronary sinus; DAo—descending aorta; IVC—inferior vena cava; IVS—interventricular septum; LA—left atrium; LPA—left pulmonary artery; LV—left ventricle; LVAW—left ventricle anterior wall; LVIW—left ventricle inferior wall; LVLW—left ventricle lateral wall; LVPW—left ventricle posterior wall; MV—mitral valve; PT—pulmonary trunk; RA—right atrium; RPA—right pulmonary artery; RV—right ventricle; RVFW—right ventricle free wall; SVC—superior vena cava; TV—tricuspid valve.

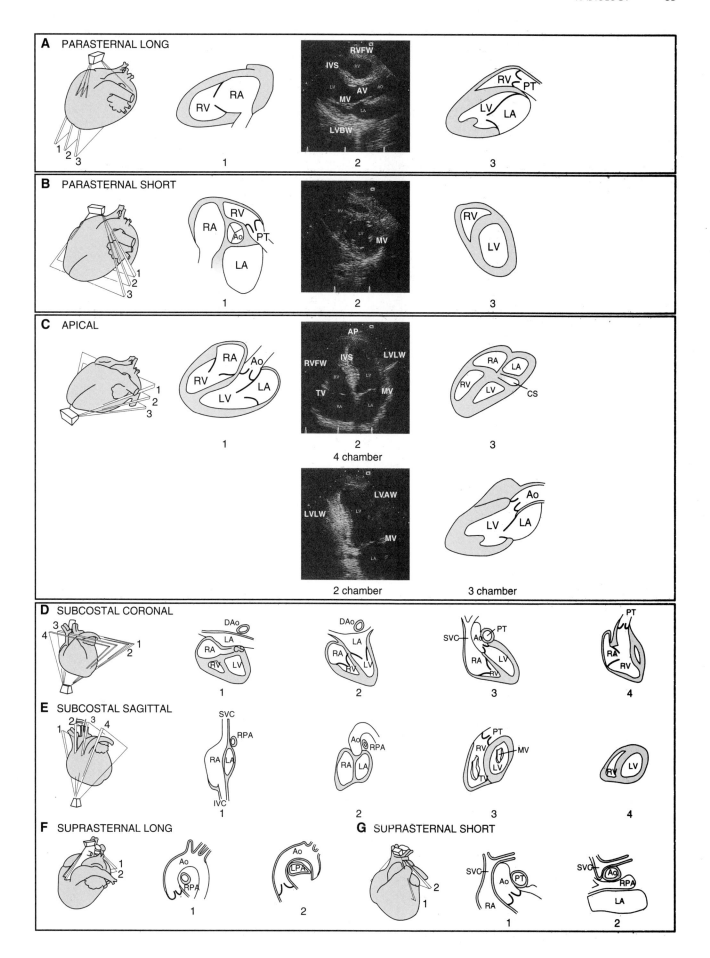

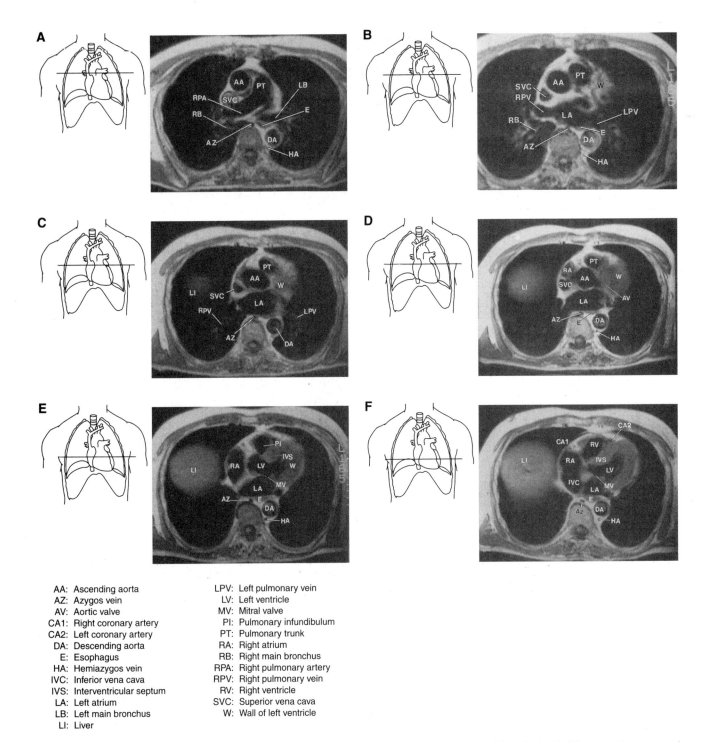

AA:	Ascending aorta
AZ:	Azygos vein
AV:	Aortic valve
CA1:	Right coronary artery
CA2:	Left coronary artery
DA:	Descending aorta
E:	Esophagus
HA:	Hemiazygos vein
IVC:	Inferior vena cava
IVS:	Interventricular septum
LA:	Left atrium
LB:	Left main bronchus
LI:	Liver
LPV:	Left pulmonary vein
LV:	Left ventricle
MV:	Mitral valve
PI:	Pulmonary infundibulum
PT:	Pulmonary trunk
RA:	Right atrium
RB:	Right main bronchus
RPA:	Right pulmonary artery
RPV:	Right pulmonary vein
RV:	Right ventricle
SVC:	Superior vena cava
W:	Wall of left ventricle

FIGURE 3-5. MRIs at six different levels. (A) At the level of the origin of the right pulmonary artery. **(B)** At the level of the ascending aorta and pulmonary trunk. **(C)** At a level just inferior to B. **(D)** At a level just inferior to C. **(E)** At a level just inferior to D. **(F)** At a level just inferior to E.

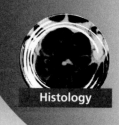

Chapter 4

Histology

❶ HEART LAYERS

The wall of the heart in all four chambers consists of three layers: **endocardium, myocardium,** and **epicardium.**

A. **Endocardium.** The endocardium is continuous with the **tunica intima** of blood vessels. The endocardium is variable in thickness: **thickest in the atria** and **thinnest in the ventricles.** The endocardium consists of: an **endothelium** (simple squamous epithelium that lines the heart chambers), a **basal lamina,** and a **layer of elastic and collagen fibers with scattered fibroblasts.** The layer of elastic and collagen fibers with scattered fibroblasts is sometimes called the **subendothelial layer.** Another layer of connective tissue, which is somewhat more dense and consists of predominantly elastic fibers, lies beneath the endocardium and is called the **subendocardial layer.** This layer is continuous with the connective tissue around the cardiac myocytes in the myocardium. It is also sometimes referred to as the **subendocardial space** because blood vessels, nerves, and Purkinje myocytes (bundle of His, right and left bundle branches) are in this space.

B. **Myocardium.** The myocardium is continuous with the **tunica media** of blood vessels. The myocardium consists of: **cardiac myocytes, myocardial endocrine cells, an intramural network of Purkinje myocytes,** and **cardiac nodal cells** (sinoatrial [SA] node and atrioventricular [AV] node).
1. **Cardiac myocytes.** Cardiac myocytes (80 µm long and 12 µm in diameter) are short, branching cylinder-shaped cells with a single centrally located nucleus. These cells are striated in appearance such that an **A band, I band, H band,** and **Z disks** can be observed. These cells have **T-tubules** (invaginations of the cell membrane at Z disks) that interact with **terminal cisternae** of the **sarcoplasmic reticulum** to form **diads.** Cardiac myocytes are joined together by **intercalated disks,** which consist of a **fascia adherens, desmosomes,** and **gap junctions.** Cardiac myocytes are *not* innervated per se (there are no neuromuscular junctions as in skeletal muscle) instead, autonomic nerve fibers **synapse en passant.** The contraction of cardiac myocytes is **"myogenic,"** which means contractions are **spontaneous** (no innervation is necessary like skeletal muscle for contraction to occur). The contraction mechanism of cardiac myocytes is similar to skeletal muscle except that cardiac myocytes use extracellular Ca^{2+} as **"trigger Ca^{2+},"** which induces more Ca^{2+} release for the sarcoplasmic reticulum. Cardiac myocytes grow by hypertrophy. Cardiac myocytes exhibit very little mitotic activity.
2. **Myocardial endocrine cells** are found in the myocardium of the right and left atria and have secretory granules containing **atrial natriuretic peptide (ANP).** ANP is secreted in response to **increased blood volume** or **increased venous pressure** within the atria (e.g., atrial distention due to left atrial failure). **ANP functions** include: increasing glomerular filtration pressure and glomerular filtration rate (via vasoconstriction of the efferent arteriole) and decreasing Na^+ reabsorption by the proximal convoluted tubule (PCT) and medullary collecting ducts. These actions produce **natriuresis** (increased Na^+ excretion) in a large volume of dilute urine; ANP inhibits secretion of **antidiuretic hormone (ADH)** from the neurohypophysis, inhibits secretion of **aldosterone** from the adrenal cortex (zona glomerulosa), inhibits secretion of **renin** from juxtaglomerular cells, and causes vasodilation of peripheral and renal blood vessels.

3. **Purkinje myocytes (PMs)** are modified cardiac myocytes that are specialized for conduction. Purkinje myocytes are **not neurons.** PMs make up the bundle of His, right and left bundle branches that travel in the subendocardial space, and then terminate as a intramural network of PMs within the myocardium. PMs are cylindrical cells that are arranged end-to-end in long rows. They are shorter than cardiac myocytes (50 μm versus 80 μm), but they have a much larger diameter than cardiac myocytes (30 μm versus 12 μm). PMs have irregular borders often with large extensions of one cell protruding into a neighboring PM that increases the surface area for cell-to-cell contact. They do not have intercalated disks; however, gap junctions are found at the ends and the sides of the cell. PMs have only scattered myofibrils, abundant mitochondria, and a high content of glycogen.

4. **Cardiac nodal cells**
   a. **Sinoatrial (SA) node or pacemaker.** The SA node (pacemaker) is located at the junction of the superior vena cava (SVC) and lateral border of the right atrium (i.e., **upper end of the crista terminalis**) just **beneath the epicardium**). The SA node is 10–15 mm long and 1–2 mm wide and is not visible to the naked eye. The SA node consists of connective tissue stroma containing an irregular whorled network of cardiac nodal cells, the SA nodal artery, and numerous nerve endings (postganglionic parasympathetic and postganglionic sympathetic). Cardiac nodal cells of the SA node are considerably smaller in diameter than cardiac myocytes (4 μm versus 12 μm). Cardiac nodal cells of the SA node are connected by **desmosomes and gap junctions** (no intercalated disks), have few myofibrils, have no organized striation pattern, have abundant mitochondria, and have some glycogen and lipid droplets.
   b. **Atrioventricular (AV) node.** The AV node is located on the right side of the interatrial septum just superior and medial to the opening of the coronary sinus just **beneath the endocardium (i.e., in the subendocardial space).** The AV node consists of connective tissue stroma containing an irregular whorled network of cardiac nodal cells, AV nodal artery, and numerous nerve endings (postganglionic parasympathetic and postganglionic sympathetic). Cardiac nodal cells of the AV node are histologically similar to cardiac nodal cells of the SA node.

C. **Epicardium.** The epicardium forms the outer covering of the heart and consists of an outer layer of simple squamous cells **(mesothelium),** which lies on a connective tissue stroma containing collagen and elastic fibers. Coronary arteries, cardiac veins, and autonomic nerve fibers travel within the epicardium. Adipocytes are also found in the epicardium. In gross anatomy, the epicardium is called the **visceral layer of serous pericardium.** At the base of the aorta and pulmonary trunk, the mesothelium of the visceral layer of serous pericardium is reflected and becomes the **parietal layer of serous pericardium.** Histologically, the visceral and parietal layers of serous pericardium are similar. They define a narrow space called the **pericardial cavity,** which contains serous fluid to lubricate the surfaces and permit friction-free movement during diastole and systole. The pericardial cavity is surrounded by the **fibrous pericardium,** which is a fairly dense layer of collagen (no elastic fibers) that is continuous with the **tunica adventitia.**

▶

FIGURE 4-1. **(A) Diagram of cardiac muscle.** Note the boundaries of the sarcomere (Z disk→Z disk), I band, the M-line bisecting the H band, and A band. The T-tubules interact with terminal cisternae of the sarcoplasmic reticulum (SR) to form a diad (*Di; circle*). T—T-tubule; mit—mitochondria. **(B) Light micrograph (LM) of cardiac myocytes in longitudinal section.** Note the intercalated disks (*arrows*) and the centrally located nuclei (*N*). **(C) LM of cardiac myocytes in cross-section.** Note the centrally located nucleus (*N, arrow*) and capillary (*cap*). **(D) Electron micrograph (EM) of cardiac myocytes in longitudinal section.** Note the centrally located nucleus (*N*), numerous mitochondria (*mit*), striations (***), and capillary (*cap*). **(E) EM of an intercalated disk in cardiac muscle.** An intercalated disk is found at the junction of two cardiac myocytes and is typically arranged in a stair-step pattern. The intercalated disk consists of a fascia adherens (*fa*), desmosomes (*des*), and gap junction (*gap*). The gap junction is always oriented parallel to the myofilaments. **(F) LM of Purkinje cells** (*P; dotted line*) traveling within the myocardium (*MY*). By light microscopy, Purkinje cells appear pale because the large amount of glycogen that is normally contained in the cytoplasm is lost during histologic processing.

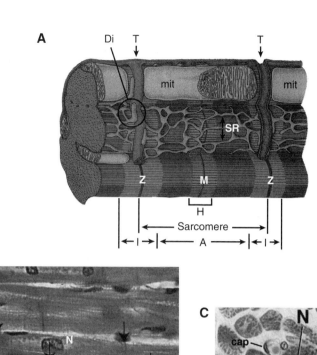

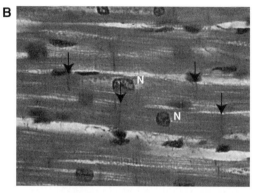

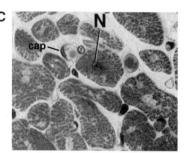

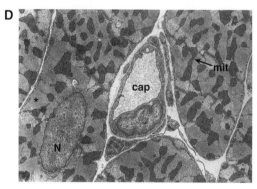

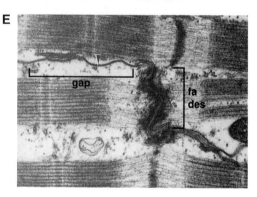

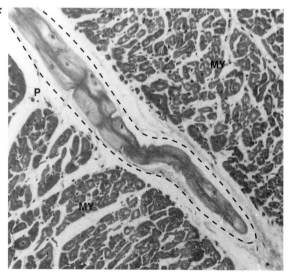

ⓘ Photomicrographs

A.   Light micrograph (LM) of cardiac muscle (longitudinal and cross-section), Electron micrograph (EM) of cardiac muscle and intercalated disk, LM of Purkinje myocytes. *(Figure 4-1)*

B.   LM of the wall of the heart. *(Figure 4-2)*

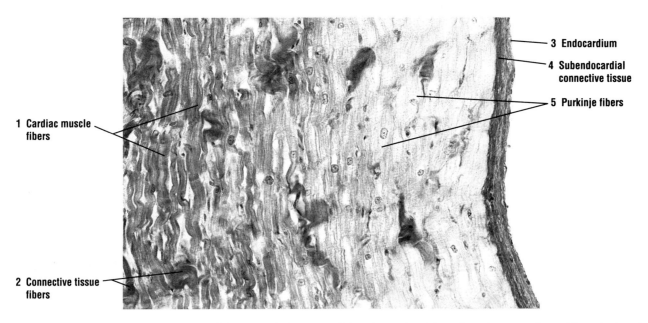

3 **Endocardium**

4 **Subendocardial connective tissue**

5 **Purkinje fibers**

1 **Cardiac muscle fibers**

2 **Connective tissue fibers**

FIGURE 4-2. Light micrograph shows the wall of the heart, which consists of three layers: the endocardium, the myocardium with predominantly contractile cardiac myocytes surrounded by connective tissue, and the epicardium (not shown).

Chapter 5

Physiology

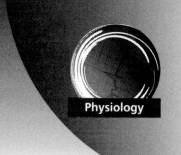

❶ Contraction of Cardiac Myocytes *(Figure 5-1).*

Cardiac muscle differs from skeletal muscle in that cardiac myocytes branch and are connected by intercalated disks to form a **syncytium.** The syncytium provides easy movement of an action potential so that when one cardiac myocyte becomes excited, the action potential spreads to all adjoining cells. The atrial syncytium is separated from the ventricular syncytium by the **fibrous skeleton** so that action potentials are conducted from the atria → ventricles only through the Purkinje system.

A. Cardiac myocytes demonstrate a **diad,** which consists of a **T tubule** located at the Z disk and flanked by one **terminal cisterna (TC).** A T tubule is an invagination of the cell membrane. A TC is a dilated sac of sarcoplasmic reticulum (SR), which stores, releases, and reaccumulates Ca^{2+}.

B. The Ca^{2+} influx that occurs at the cell membrane and T tubule in **phase 2** of the action potential through L-type Ca^{2+} channels is *not* sufficient to cause contraction but acts as **trigger Ca^{2+}** that stimulates release of a large pool of Ca^{2+} stored in TC **(i.e., intracellular Ca^{2+} increases).**

C. Ca^{2+} binds to **troponin C,** which allows the **myosin crossbridge-ADP-PO_4^{2-}** complex to bind actin. From this point on, cardiac myocyte contraction resembles skeletal muscle contraction.

D. $ADP + PO_4^{2-}$ is released, leaving the myosin crossbridge bound to actin. Thick and thin filaments slide past each other **(i.e., power stroke). The magnitude of the force of contraction is proportional to the intracellular Ca^{2+}.**

E. The myosin crossbridge binds adenosine 5′-triphosphate (ATP), which detaches the myosin crossbridge from actin.

F. ATP hydrolysis occurs by **myosin ATPase** and the products ($ADP + PO_4^{2-}$) remain bound to the myosin crossbridge, thereby reforming the myosin crossbridge-ADP-PO_4^{2-} complex.

G. As Ca^{2+} influx begins to decrease at the end of phase 2, Ca^{2+} is pumped from the cytoplasm back into the TC/SR by **Ca^{2+} ATPase** that is regulated by an intramembranous SR protein called **phospholamban (i.e., relaxation).**

H. Troponin C is freed of Ca^{2+}.

I. The phases of contraction of the entire heart are called **systole** (the period during which cardiac contraction occurs) and **diastole** (the period during which cardiac relaxation and filling occurs. The heart chambers fill during diastole so that the volume of blood in the heart is greatest at the end of diastole. The thickness of the heart walls is indicative of the work they must do to pump blood into their respective circulations. The pressure in the systemic circulation is significantly higher than that of the pulmonary circulation, although the blood flow through both is equal. Therefore, the wall of the left ventricle is much thicker than that of the right ventricle to overcome the higher pressure in the systemic circulation.

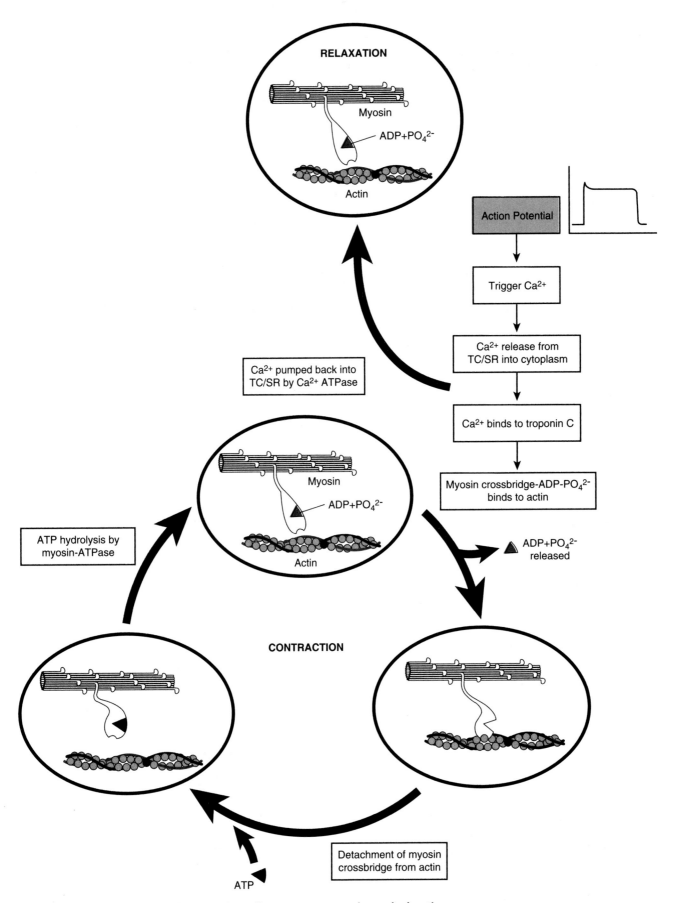

FIGURE 5-1. **Diagram indicating the events in cardiac myocyte contraction and relaxation.**

Preload

Preload is the load on ventricular myocytes at the end of diastole. Therefore, preload is the load on the heart before contraction. The preload of the right ventricle and the preload of the left ventricle are equal. The best index of preload is **end-diastolic volume,** which is the volume of blood contained in the left ventricle at the end of diastole or just before contraction. **Pulmonary artery wedge pressure** measured by a Swan-Ganz catheter is another index used clinically because of ease of measurement.

A. **Factors that increase preload**
   1. **Overinfusion of saline**
   2. **Edema**
   3. **Exercise**

B. **Factor that decreases preload.** Venous dilation (e.g., nitroglycerin, isosorbide dinitrate [Isordil Sorbitrate]), amyl nitrite [Aspirols]). These drugs relax predominantly **venous** smooth muscle leading to peripheral venous dilation via the active metabolite **nitric oxide (NO),** which activates guanylate cyclase and **increases guanosine** 3′, 5′-cyclic monophosphate (cGMP). The increase in cGMP causes dephosphorylation of myosin light chains.

 Afterload

Afterload is the load on ventricular myocytes during contraction. Therefore, afterload is the magnitude of load the heart must overcome to eject blood. The best index of afterload is **aortic pressure** (for left ventricle) and **pulmonary artery pressure** (for right ventricle).

A. **Factor that increases afterload.** Arteriolar constriction (e.g., hypertension)

B. **Factors that decrease afterload**
   1. **Vasodilators (e.g., hydralazine [Apresoline], minoxidil [Loniten]).** These drugs relax predominantly **arteriolar** smooth muscle, leading to a decrease in peripheral vascular resistance (PVR). The action of hydralazine is uncertain but may involve NO. Minoxidil is a K$^+$ channel agonist that causes an increased K$^+$ efflux, hyperpolarization, and relaxation of smooth muscle.
   2. **Angiotensin-converting enzyme (ACE) inhibitors (e.g., captopril [Capoten], enalapril [Vasotec], lisinopril [Zestril]).** These drugs reversibly inhibit ACE, thereby preventing the conversion of angiotensin I to angiotensin II (a potent vasoconstrictor).
   3. **Angiotensin II receptor antagonist (e.g., losartan [Cozaar]).** This drug blocks the angiotensin II receptor.

IV **Contractility (Inotropism) and Frank-Starling Curve** *(Figure 5-2A)*

Contractility is the force of contraction of ventricular myocytes at a given muscle length (preload), which is classically described by the **Frank-Starling curve (or cardiac function curve).** Therefore, contractility is an index that measures the ability of the heart to pump blood. The Frank-Starling law indicates that as cardiac muscle is stretched, its ability to contract is augmented. This means that when an additional amount of blood returns to the ventricles, the ventricles are stretched; the result is augmented contraction that propels the additional blood out of the ventricles. This ensures that both ventricles pump the same volume of blood within one heartbeat, thereby preventing any overfilling of the pulmonary or systemic circulations. The best clinical index of contractility is **ejection fraction (EF),** defined as the percentage of blood pumped by the heart on each beat. The EF stroke volume/end-diastolic volume it is normally **55%.**

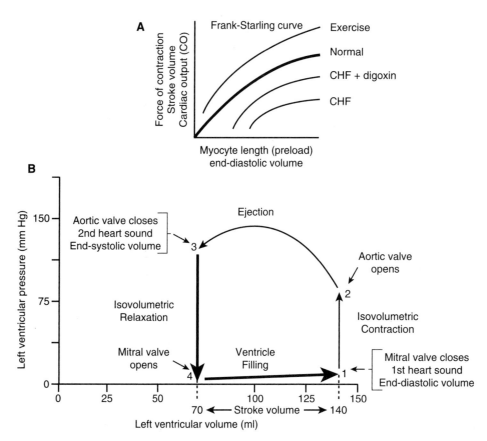

	Increase	Decrease
Preload	• Overinfusion of saline • Edema • Exercise	• Venous dilation (nitroglycerin, isosorbide, dinitrate, amyl nitrate)
Afterload	• Arteriolar constriction (hypertension)	• Vasodilators (hydralazine, minoxidil) • ACE Inhibitors (captopril, enalapril, lisinopril) • Angiotensin II receptor antagonists (losartan)
Contractility	• Increased heart rate (Bowditch staircase) • Sympathetic stimulation (catecholamines, dobutamine) • Cardiac glycosides (digoxin, digitoxin)	• Heart failure • Acidosis • Hypoxia/Hypercapnea • Parasympathetic stimulation (ACh) • β_1-adrenergic antagonist (metoprolol)

A. **Factors that increase contractility (positive inotropism)**

1. **Increased heart rate (Bowditch staircase phenomenon)** strengthens the force of contraction in a stepwise fashion as intracellular Ca^{2+} is elevated cumulatively over several heartbeats.

2. **Sympathetic stimulation (e.g., catecholamines via β_1-adrenergic receptor, dobutamine [Dobutrex]).** Dobutamine is a β_1-adrenergic agonist.

3. **Cardiac glycosides (e.g. digoxin [Lanoxin] and digitoxin [Crystodigin]).** These drugs are Na^+-K^+ ATPase blockers that elevate intracellular Na^+. The elevated Na^+ overwhelms the Na^+-Ca^{2+} exchanger so that more Ca^{2+} can be reaccumulated by terminal cisternae (TCs). During the next contraction, more Ca^{2+} is released from TCs, increasing the force of contraction.

B. **Factors that decrease contractility (negative inotropism)**

1. **Heart failure**
2. **Acidosis**
3. **Hypoxia/hypercapnia**
4. **Parasympathetic stimulation (e.g., acetylcholine [Ach] via M_2 muscarinic ACh receptor).** See Chapter 4 IV
5. **β_1-adrenergic antagonist (e.g., metoprolol [Lopressor])**

 Swan-Ganz Catheter

A Swan-Ganz catheter is a relatively soft, flexible right heart catheter with an inflatable balloon at its tip. The balloon allows the catheter to float through the right heart chambers and into the pulmonary artery before "wedging" in a distal branch of the pulmonary artery. The information gained from a Swan-Ganz catheter is as follows:

A. **Cardiac output (CO)** is measured by the thermodilution technique.

B. **Pulmonary artery wedge pressure (PAWP)** is obtained by inflating the balloon while the catheter is positioned in a distal branch of the pulmonary artery. This shields the catheter tip from the proximal pressure in the pulmonary artery proximally, so that the distal pressure in the pulmonary arterioles can be measured (PAWP). PAWP approximates the pressure in the left atrium. Assuming no obstruction between the left atrium and the left ventricle, PAWP approximates the *left ventricle* end-diastolic *pressure* (LVEDP). The LVEDP is the clinical measure of left ventricle **(LV) preload.** Technically, LV end-diastolic volume determines LV preload (not pressure), but LV end-diastolic volume is very difficult to measure.

◄

FIGURE 5-2. **(A) The Frank-Starling curve or cardiac function curve.** Note the relationship of the force of contraction to myocyte length (preload). In the ventricle, stroke volume (SV) is a good indicator of force of contraction and end-diastolic volume is a good indicator of myocyte length. Note that as the end-diastolic volume (or venous return) increases, the SV increases. Note the changes in the curve due to congestive heart failure (CHF), CHF plus treatment with digoxin, and exercise. **(B)** Left ventricular pressure-volume curve through one cardiac cycle. Thin lines (1 → 2 and 2 → 3) indicate the **systolic portion** of the curve. Thick lines (3 → 4 and 4 → 1) indicate the **diastolic portion** of the curve. Note the events at points 1, 2, 3, and 4 as indicated by the *arrows*. Beginning at point 1, the left ventricle begins to contract, which leads to mitral valve closure. However, the aortic valve has not yet opened so that the **period 1 → 2 is the isovolumetric ventricular contraction phase.** At point 2, the aortic valve opens when sufficient pressure has been generated to overcome aortic pressure, and blood is pumped from the ventricle into the aorta. The **period 2 → 3 is the rapid and reduced ventricular ejection phase.** The amount of blood ejected during period 2 → 3 is called the **stroke volume** (140 mL − 70 mL = 70 mL). At point 3, the left ventricle begins to relax and the pressure falls rapidly resulting in closure of the aortic valve. The mitral valve remains closed until point 4. The **period 3 → 4 is the isovolumetric ventricular relaxation phase.** At point 4, the mitral valve opens to permit ventricular filling when left atrial pressure exceeds left ventricular pressure. The **period 4 → 1 is the rapid and reduced ventricular filling phase.** **(C)** Left ventricular pressure-volume curve depicting an increase in preload (*dotted line*). Note the **shift to the right** of the curve and the **increase in SV. (D)** Left ventricular pressure-volume curve depicting an increase in afterload (*dotted line*). Note the increase in **left ventricle pressure** and **decrease in SV. (E)** Left ventricular pressure-volume curve depicting an increase in contractility (*dotted line*). Note the **increase in SV** and **no change in end-diastolic volume. (F)** Left ventricular pressure-volume curve depicting a decrease in contractility (*dotted line*). Note the **decrease in SV** and **increase in end-systolic volume.**

C. **CO and PAWP** are important physiological parameters to measure with the Swan-Ganz catheter because they allow the physician to apply the Frank-Starling law, which states that an increase in preload (PAWP) produces an increase in CO at any given level of myocardial contractility.

D. **Pulmonary artery pressure** is measured when the balloon is deflated.

E. **Right atrium pressure** is measured using a port 15 cm proximal to the catheter tip. This port is also used to infuse drugs or fluids into the central circulation.

F. **Mixed venous oxyhemoglobin saturation (SvO₂)** is measured using fiberoptics.

VI Left Ventricle Pressure–Volume Curves *(Figure 5-2B–F)*

The events of the cardiac cycle can be summarized by the relation between left ventricular pressure and left ventricular volume. The effects of preload, afterload, and contractility can also be graphically depicted using the pressure-volume curve.

A

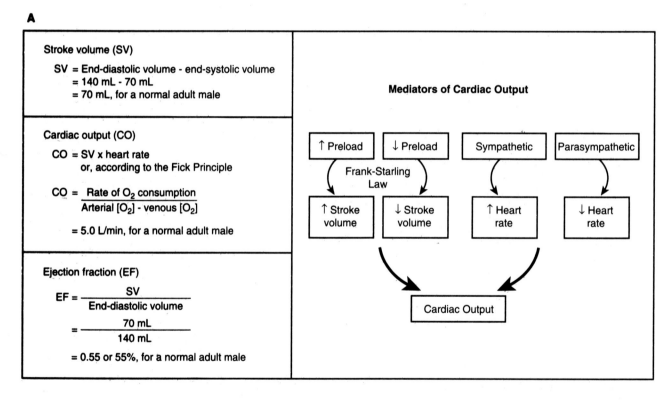

B

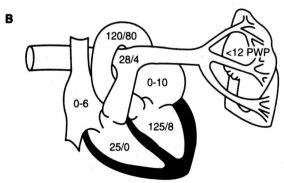

Ⅶ Cardiac Calculations *(Figure 5-3A)*

A. **Stroke volume (SV)** is the volume of blood ejected from the ventricle on each heartbeat.

B. **Cardiac output** is the stroke volume multiplied by the heart rate.

C. **Ejection fraction (EF)** is the fraction of the end-diastolic volume ejected in each **SV**.

Ⅷ Pressures Within Heart Chambers and Great Vessels *(Figure 5-3B)*

A. **Right atrium (0–6 mm Hg; median 4 mm Hg).** The right atrium is a very compliant chamber that holds blood as it moves from the systemic circulation to return to the heart. Because of its high degree of compliance and weak contraction, the pressure within the right atrium undergoes little change. As the right atrium fills with blood, the pressure rises from **0 to 6 mm Hg,** with a mean pressure of about **4 mm Hg.**

B. **Right ventricle (25/0 mm Hg).** The right ventricle pumps blood into the pulmonary artery and has pressures ranging from **25 mm Hg systolic to 0 mm Hg diastolic.**

C. **Pulmonary artery (28/4 mm Hg).** The pressure within the pulmonary artery ranges from **28 mm Hg systolic to 4 mm Hg diastolic.**

D. **Left atrium (0–10 mm Hg; 8 mm Hg).** The left atrium receives blood returning from the pulmonary circulation and has pressure ranging from **0–10 mm Hg** with a mean pressure of about **8 mm Hg.**

E. **Left ventricle (125/8 mm Hg).** The left ventricle pumps blood into the aorta and has pressures ranging from **125 mm Hg systolic to 8 mm Hg diastolic.**

F. **Aorta (120/80 mm Hg).** The pressure within the **aorta** ranges from **120 mm Hg systolic to 80 mm Hg diastolic.**

Ⅸ The Cardiac Cycle *(Figure 5-4A)*

The cardiac cycle includes both **electrical events** of the heart (measured by electrocardiogram [ECG]) and **mechanical events** associated with the contraction and relaxation of the heart. A cardiac cycle refers to the period from the start of one heartbeat through the start of the next heartbeat. A cardiac cycle is divided into seven phases. Key points in each phase are indicated below.

A. **Atrial systole.** The **P wave** initiates atrial systole and ejects more blood into the ventricles. Atrial systole generates the ***a* wave,** which is reflected back into the large veins and may be recorded from the jugular vein. The appearance of **distended jugular veins** in a patient indicates excessive pressure in the right atrium, which may be

◀

FIGURE 5-3. (A) Calculations of stroke volume (*SV*), cardiac output (*CO*), and ejection fraction (*EF*). A flow chart of the key mediators of CO is shown. Note that CO is affected by both SV and heart rate (i.e., CO = SV × heart rate). This indicates that an increase (or decrease) in either SV or heart rate will increase (or decrease) CO. What causes an increase (or decrease) in SV? The SV is determined primarily by the preload as defined by the Frank-Starling law, which indicates that as preload increases, the SV increases until the SV reaches a plateau. In addition, as the preload decreases, the SV decreases. What causes an increase (or decrease) in heart rate? The heart rate is determined primarily by the sympathetic innervation (increases heart rate) and the parasympathetic innervation (decreases heart rate). If heart rate increases, then CO increases. If heart rate decreases, then CO decreases. However, when the heart rate increases to > 150 beats/min, CO decreases because the SV decreases significantly. At > 150 beats/min, the SV decreases because the heart spends less time in diastole, and therefore the time available for the rapid and reduced ventricular filling phase of the cardiac cycle is decreased. If the heart fills with less blood, the preload is reduced, which affects the SV. **(B) Diagram of normal blood pressures (mm Hg; systole/diastole) within heart chambers and great vessels.** Note that pulmonary wedge pressure (*PWP*) measured with a Swan-Ganz catheter is a good estimate of left atrial pressure (< 12 mm Hg).

A The Cardiac Cycle

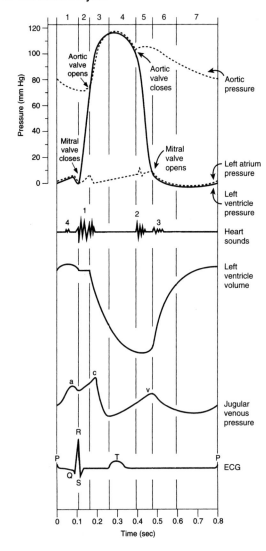

B Aortic Valve Insufficiency

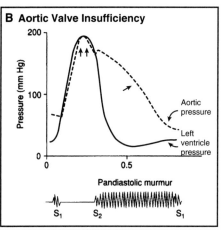

C Mitral Valve Stenosis

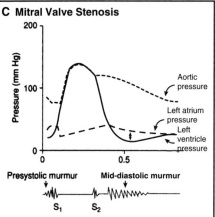

D Aortic Valve Stenosis

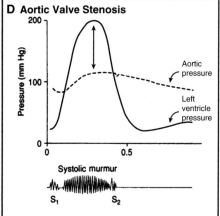

E Mitral Valve Insufficiency

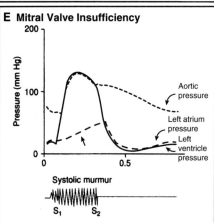

caused by congestive heart failure (CHF) or tricuspid valve dysfunction. Atrial systole contributes (but is not essential for) ventricle filling and causes S_4, which is not audible in normal adults.

B. **Isovolumetric ventricular contraction.** After the onset of the **QRS complex,** the ventricles begin to contract and the ventricular pressure begins to rise. As the ventricular pressure exceeds atrial pressure, the atrioventricular (AV) valves (mitral and tricuspid) close. Closure of the AV valves causes S_1. The mitral valve closes before the tricuspid valve so that S_1 may be split **(S_1 splitting).** Note that during this phase, even though the ventricles contract, there is no change in blood volume (i.e., isovolumetric) because **all the valves are closed** (mitral, tricuspid, aortic, and pulmonic).

C. **Rapid ventricular ejection.** When ventricular pressure exceeds the pressure within the aorta and pulmonary artery, the **aortic valve and pulmonic valve open,** respectively. Right ventricular ejection occurs before left ventricular ejection because the pressure is lower in the pulmonary artery than in the aorta. **A majority of the stroke volume is ejected** during this phase. The **T wave** marks the end of the rapid ventricular ejection phase. Note that **atrial filling** begins during this phase.

D. **Reduced ventricular ejection.** During this phase, ventricular pressure begins to decrease while ejection of blood from the ventricles continues but is slower. The pressure within the aorta and pulmonary artery decreases as blood flows from the large arteries into smaller arteries. Atrial filling continues.

E. **Isovolumetric ventricular relaxation.** Since the **T wave** has already been completed, the ventricles are now repolarized. The aortic valve and pulmonic valve close, which produces S_2. Normally, the aortic valve closes first, producing the aortic component of S_2 called A_2. Then, the pulmonic valve closes producing the pulmonic component of S_2 called P_2. During this phase, ventricular pressure decreases rapidly. Note also that during this phase there is no change in blood volume (i.e., isovolumetric) because **all the valves are closed** (mitral, tricuspid, aortic, and pulmonic). However, when the ventricular

◄

FIGURE 5-4. (A) The cardiac cycle. The events in the cardiac cycle are summarized for the left side of the heart. Similar events occur for the right side of the heart, although the pressures are reduced. The seven phases (1–7) of the cardiac cycle are separated by the vertical lines. 1: atrial systole; 2: isovolumetric ventricular contraction; 3: rapid ventricular ejection; 4: reduced ventricular ejection; 5: isovolumetric ventricular relaxation; 6: rapid ventricular filling; 7: reduced ventricular filling. Use the ECG as an event marker and note how the jugular venous pressure, left ventricle volume, heart sounds, left ventricle pressure, left atrium pressure, and aortic pressure change during the ECG. **Jugular venous pressure:** The a wave is produced by right atrial systole. The a wave increases in amplitude as the vigor of atrial systole increases. A giant a wave (called a **cannon wave**) is observed when the right atrium contracts against a closed tricuspid valve. The **c wave** is produced by right ventricle systole (i.e., the tricuspid valve bulging into atrium). The **v wave** is produced by an increase in right atrial pressure due to filling against closed tricuspid valve. The v wave terminates when the tricuspid valve opens. P—P wave; QRS—QRS complex; T—T wave. **(B) Aortic valve insufficiency.** In this case, the aortic semilunar valve does not close properly at the beginning of diastole such that a regurgitation of blood from the aorta to the left ventricle occurs, producing a **diastolic murmur (i.e., pandiastolic because it lasts throughout diastole).** The amount of blood regurgitated into the left ventricle may be as high as 60–70% of the amount ejected during systole. The regurgitation of blood causes a **low aortic diastolic pressure** (arrow). In addition, the regurgitation of blood augments the next stroke volume, resulting in a **high aortic systolic pressure** (double arrow). Note also the high ventricular systolic pressure ($\approx$ 200 mm Hg). The pulse pressure may also be extremely high (called **Corrigan's water-hammer pulses**), which may be detectable in the nail beds. This condition produces marked left ventricle dilation, which eventually leads to left ventricle failure. **(C) Mitral valve stenosis.** In this case, a narrow mitral valve orifice impedes blood flow from the left atrium into the left ventricle during diastole such that a pressure gradient between the left atrium and left ventricle develops (arrow), producing **diastolic murmurs.** The diastolic murmur that occurs during atrial systole is called the **presystolic murmur.** The diastolic murmur that occurs during the rapid filling phase is called the **mid-diastolic murmur.** These two murmurs are often described as the **crescendo murmur** and **decrescendo murmur,** respectively. The stenosis causes extremely high pressure and volume in the left atrium. This leads to pulmonary edema, enlargement of the left atrium, and atrial fibrillation. **(D) Aortic valve stenosis.** In this case, a narrow aortic valve orifice impedes the blood flow from the left ventricle into the aorta producing a **systolic murmur.** The murmur increases in loudness as systole progresses, and its duration correlates with severity of the aortic valve stenosis. A left ventricular systolic pressure that is much higher than the aortic systolic pressure is pathognomonic of aortic valve stenosis (arrow). **(E) Mitral valve insufficiency.** In this case, the mitral valve does not close properly such that a regurgitation of blood from the left ventricle to the left atrium occurs during ventricular systole, producing a **systolic murmur.** The murmur is an evenly pitched sound ("blowing") that continues through all or part of systole. The insufficiency causes high pressure and volume in the left atrium (arrow).

pressure falls below the atrial pressure, the **AV valves open.** A "blip" in aortic pressure (called the **dicrotic notch**) occurs after closure of the aortic valve.

F.   Rapid ventricular filling. Rapid ventricular filling begins as the AV valves open. The flow of blood from the atria to the ventricles produces S_3. Pressure within the aorta and pulmonary artery continues to decrease as blood continues to flow from the large arteries into smaller arteries.

G.   Reduced ventricular filling (diastasis). Filling of the ventricles continues, but at a slower rate. This is the longest phase of the cardiac cycle. Note that the time required for rapid ventricular filling and diastasis depends on the heart rate. The faster the heart rate, the shorter time available for ventricle filling.

Ⓧ Heart Sounds

A. S_1 is due to mitral and tricuspid valve closure during early systole. Even though S_1 is due to two valve closures, it is normally heard through the stethoscope as a single high-frequency sound.

B. S_2 is due to aortic and pulmonic valve closure. During normal expiration, S_2 is heard as a single sound. During normal inspiration, S_2 becomes audibly split into the aortic component (A_2) and pulmonic component (P_2), which is called **normal splitting of S_2.** Pathologically (e.g., aortic stenosis, left bundle branch block), the separation between A_2 and P_2 *decreases* during inspiration, which is called **paradoxical splitting of S_2.**

C. S_3 is due to the flow of blood from the atria to the ventricles as the mitral and tricuspid valve open during early diastole (start of rapid ventricle filling). S_3 is heard as a dull, low-pitched sound with the bell of the stethoscope placed at the cardiac apex with the patient in the left lateral decubitus position. The presence of S_3 in children and young adults is normal. However, S_3 in older adults indicates CHF. A pathological S_3 is referred to as **ventricular gallop.**

D. S_4 is due to filling of ventricle by atrial systole. S_4 becomes more forceful and more easily audible when filling is against a "stiffened" ventricle". Hence, S_4 is an indicator of cardiac disease (e.g., myocardial infarction, hypertension, and aortic stenosis). S_4 is heard as a dull, low-pitched sound with the bell of the stethoscope placed at the cardiac apex with the patient in the left lateral decubitus position (in the case of left-sided S_4). S_4 is referred to as **atrial gallop.**

Ⓧ︎Ⓘ Heart Murmurs *(Figure 5-4 B–E)*

Heart murmurs are important physical signs of valve lesions. Murmurs are caused by either turbulent blood flow or changes in direction of blood flow.

A.   Pathological diastolic murmurs. In contrast to systolic murmurs, diastolic murmurs are seldom innocent. The most common pathological diastolic murmurs are due to the following:

   1.   Aortic valve insufficiency and pulmonic valve insufficiency. The insufficiency of the aortic or pulmonic valves allows mild degrees of blood regurgitation across these valves. This produces a diastolic murmur that is termed **pandiastolic** because it lasts throughout diastole. These two pathologies are the most common causes of a diastolic murmur.

   2.   Mitral valve stenosis. A narrow mitral valve impedes blood flow from the left atrium into the left ventricle. This produces **diastolic murmurs.** The diastolic murmur that occurs during atrial systole is called the **presystolic murmur.** The diastolic murmur that occurs during the rapid filling phase is called the **mid-diastolic murmur.** These two murmurs are often described as the **crescendo and decrescendo murmurs,** respectively.

B. **Innocent systolic murmurs** include the following:
   1. **Still's (vibratory) murmur** is described by its musical sound of "vibration," "groaning," or "twanging" and is the most common innocent murmur in children 3 to 6 years of age.
   2. **Pulmonary flow murmur** is described as an early to midsystolic, crescendo–decrescendo murmur.
   3. **Neonatal physiological peripheral pulmonary artery stenosis murmur** is frequently present in newborns, begins in early to midsystole, and radiates to the infraclavicular area, axilla, and back. This murmur subsides within the first year of life.
   4. **Aortic systolic murmur** is described as systolic ejection flow murmur heard maximally in the aortic area.
   5. **Supraclavicular murmur** is described as a low-pitched systolic murmur maximally audible above the clavicles and radiates to the neck bilaterally. It is heard in children and young adults.

C. **Pathological systolic murmurs.** The most common pathological systolic murmurs are due to the following:
   1. **Aortic valve stenosis** produces a harsh, often noisy, murmur best heard in the right upper sternal border. This murmur increases in loudness as systole progresses, and its duration correlates with the severity of the aortic stenosis.
   2. **Mitral valve insufficiency** produces an evenly pitched sound ("blowing") best heard at the cardiac apex and may radiate to the left axilla. This murmur continues through all or part of systole.
   3. **Tricuspid valve insufficiency** produces an evenly pitched sound ("blowing") best heard at the lower left sternal border. This murmur continues through all or part of systole and increases with inspiration.
   4. **Hypertrophic cardiomyopathy** produces a not very loud or harsh sound best heard at the mid-left sternal border. This murmur is a widely split and fixed S_2 that does not vary with respiration.
   5. **Atrial septal defect (ASD)** produces a not very loud or harsh sound best heard at the upper portion of intercostal space 2.
   6. **Ventricular septal defect (VSD)** produces a loud, harsh sound best heard at the left sternal border at intercostal space 3 or 4.

XII Myogenic Heartbeat

Cardiac myocytes contract through intrinsically generated action potentials, which are then passed on to neighboring myocytes by gap junctions; that is, the heartbeat is myogenic. The spontaneous, intrinsically generated action potentials are due to the expression of genes that code for various ion channel proteins and carrier (or transporter) proteins that get inserted into the myocyte cell membrane and begin the flux of ions. This flux of ions generates the action potential. There are two types of action potentials.

A. **Slow-response action potentials** (*Figure 5-5A*). Slow-response action potentials are observed in the **sinoatrial (SA) node** and **AV node.** They are due to the presence of **slow (funny) Na⁺ channels** and are divided into three phases only, as indicated below.
   1. **Phase 0** is due to the **Ca^{2+} influx** into nodal cells through **L-type Ca^{2+} channels** (long-lasting voltage-gated channel).
   2. **Phase 3** is due to the **K⁺ efflux** through **K⁺ channels** out of nodal cells.

A Slow

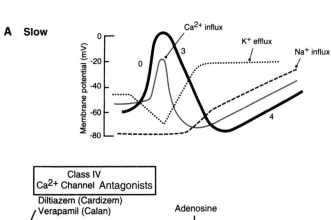

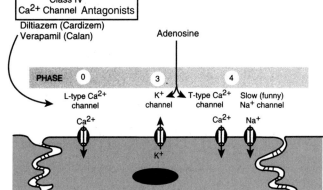

Class IV
Ca^{2+} Channel Antagonists

Diltiazem (Cardizem)
Verapamil (Calan)

Adenosine

PHASE	0	3	4
	L-type Ca^{2+} channel	K$^+$ channel	T-type Ca^{2+} channel	Slow (funny) Na$^+$ channel

B Fast

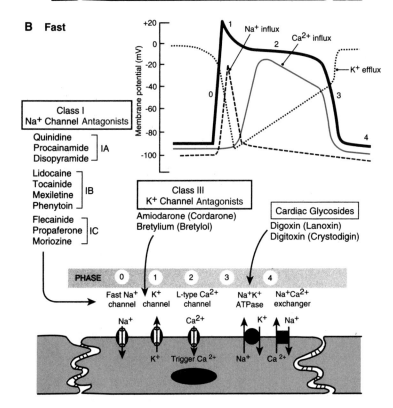

Class I
Na$^+$ Channel Antagonists

Quinidine
Procainamide   ] IA
Disopyramide

Lidocaine
Tocainide
Mexiletine   ] IB
Phenytoin

Flecainide
Propaferone   ] IC
Moriozine

Class III
K$^+$ Channel Antagonists

Amiodarone (Cordarone)
Bretylium (Bretylol)

Cardiac Glycosides

Digoxin (Lanoxin)
Digitoxin (Crystodigin)

PHASE	0	1	2	3	4
	Fast Na$^+$ channel	K$^+$ channel	L-type Ca^{2+} channel	Na$^+$K$^+$ ATPase	Na$^+$Ca^{2+} exchanger

C

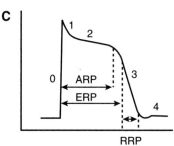

3. **Phase 4** is due to the **Ca^{2+} influx** into nodal cells through **T-type Ca^{2+} channels** (transient voltage-gated channel) and **Na^+ influx** into nodal cells through **slow (funny) Na^+ channels.** Note that phase 4 is a gradual depolarization.

B. **Fast-response action potentials** (*Figure 5-5B*). Fast-response action potentials are observed in the **atrial myocytes, bundle of His, Purkinje myocytes,** and **ventricular myocytes.** They are due to the presence of **fast Na^+ channels** and are divided into five phases.
   1. **Phase 0** is due to Na^+ **influx** into cardiac myocytes through **fast Na^+ channels.**
   2. **Phase 1** is due to **inactivation of fast Na^+ channels** and **K^+ efflux** out of cardiac myocytes through **K^+ channels.**
   3. **Phase 2** is due to **Ca^{2+} influx** into cardiac myocytes through **L-type Ca^{2+} channels.** This Ca^{2+} influx (called trigger Ca^{2+}) is involved in the contraction of cardiac myocytes.
   4. **Phase 3** is due to **inactivation of Ca^{2+} channels** and **K^+ efflux** out of cardiac myocytes through K^+ channels.
   5. **Phase 4** is due to **high K^+ efflux, removal of the excess Na^+** that entered in phase 0 by **Na^+-K^+ ATPase,** and **removal of the excess Ca^{2+}** that entered in phase 2 by the **Na^+-Ca^{2+} exchanger.**

XIII Parasympathetic (Cranial Nerve) Regulation of Heart Rate (*Figure 5-6*)

The **effects of the parasympathetic nervous system on the heart** include:

A. **Decreases heart rate** ("vagal arrest") by decreasing Na^+ influx associated with phase 4 depolarization in nodal tissue. This is also called a **negative chronotropism.**

B. **Decreases conduction velocity through the AV node (i.e., increases PR interval)** by decreasing Ca^{2+} influx associated with phase 0 depolarization in nodal tissue. This is also called a **negative dromotropism.**

C. **Decreases contractility of atrial myocytes** by decreasing Ca^{2+} influx associated with phase 2 in atrial myocytes. This is also called a **negative inotropism.**

◄

FIGURE 5-5. (A) Slow-response action potential and associated ion fluxes observed in the sinoatrial node (SA) and atrioventricular (AV) node. **Class IV Ca^{2+} channel antagonists** (diltiazem and verapamil) block L-type Ca^{2+} channels. **Adenosine** binds to adenosine receptors, which results in the activation of K^+ channels and inhibits T-type Ca^{2+} channels. **Note that phase 0 is due to Ca^{2+} influx. (B)** Fast-response action potential and associated ion fluxes observed in atrial myocytes, bundle of His, Purkinje myocytes, and ventricular myocytes. Various **antiarrhythmic drugs** are indicated along with their specific effect on ion channels. **Class I Na^+ channel antagonists** include: class IA, IB, and IC. **Class IA** (quinidine, procainamide, disopyramide) blocks open Na^+ channels. **Class IB** (lidocaine, tocainide, mexiletine, phenytoin) blocks open and closed Na^+ channels. **Class IC** (flecainide, propafenone, moricizine) blocks Na^+ channels. **Class III K^+ channel antagonists** (amiodarone and bretylium) block K^+ channels. **Cardiac glycosides** (digoxin and digitoxin) are Na^+-K^+ ATPase antagonists that elevate intracellular Na^+. The elevated Na^+ overwhelms the Na^+-Ca^{2+} exchanger so that more Ca^{2+} can be reaccumulated by terminal cisternae (TCs). During the next contraction, more Ca^{2+} ions are released from TCs, increasing the force of contraction. Cardiac glycosides are used in congestive heart failure to increase the strength of contraction. The antiarrhythmic effect of cardiac glycosides is due to their indirect effect on the autonomic nervous system (increase parasympathetic activity and decrease sympathetic activity). **Note that phase 0 is due to Na^+ influx and the long plateau (phase 1 and phase 2) of about 300 msec. (C) Refractory periods.** Compared with action potentials in neurons or skeletal muscle, the fast-response action potential in cardiac muscle is much longer in duration, which results in a prolonged refractory period. A refractory period (about 250 msec) is the time at which a cardiac myocyte cell cannot be restimulated. A prolonged refractory period is necessary in cardiac myocytes to permit the ventricles sufficient time to empty their blood volume and refill with blood before the next contraction. The degree of refraction reflects the number of fast Na^+ channels that have recovered and are capable of reopening during phase 3. The **absolute refractory period (ARP)** refers to the time during which a cardiac myocyte is **completely unexcitable** in response to a new stimulation. The **effective refractory period (ERP)** refers to a short time past the ARP during which a cardiac myocyte cell produces a **localized action potential that does not propagate** in response to a new stimulation. The **relative refractory period (RRP)** refers to the time interval during which a cardiac myocyte produces an action potential that is propagated; however, because the cardiac myocyte is stimulated at a voltage less negative than the resting potential, the upstroke of the action potential (phase 0) is less steep and of lower amplitude. During RRP, a larger-than-normal stimulus is needed to cause an action potential.

ⅩⅣ Sympathetic Regulation of Heart Rate *(Figure 5-6)*

The **effects of the sympathetic nervous system on the heart** include:

A. **Increases heat rate** by increasing Na^+ influx associated with phase 4 depolarization in nodal tissue. This is also called **positive chronotropism.**

B. **Increases conduction velocity through the AV node (i.e., increases PR interval)** by increasing Ca^{2+} influx associated with phase 0 in nodal tissue. This is also called **positive dromotropism.**

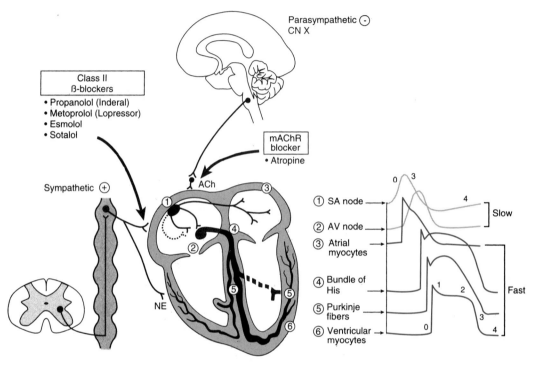

ECG	Heart Action
P wave	Represents atrial depolarization (0.08–0.1 sec)
PR interval	Is the interval from start of atrial depolarization to the start of ventricle depolarization (0.12-0.20 sec)
	Gets shorter as the heart rate increases
	Gets longer as conduction velocity through AV node is slowed (e.g., heart block)
QRS complex	Represents ventricle depolarization (0.06-0.10 sec)
QT interval	Represents the entire period of ventricle depolarization and ventricle repolarization (0.32 sec)
ST segment	Represents the period when the entire ventricle is depolarized
T wave	Represents ventricle repolarization (0.1–0.25 sec)

5 mm = 0.5 mV
1 mm = 0.1 mV

5 mm = 0.2 sec
(1 mm = 1 small box = 0.04 sec)

Paper speed: 25 mm/sec

FIGURE 5-6. Diagram of the conduction system of the heart. Action potentials from various areas of the heart are shown. The ECG is a record of the electrical activation of the heart and is the body surface manifestation of all these action potentials (1–6). As a wave of depolarization progresses through the heart, the area (outside the depolarized cardiac muscle cell) becomes electrically negative relative to areas not yet depolarized. This makes the heart a dipole or an electrical source consisting of asymmetrically distributed electrical charges. Because of the ions present in body fluids and other body structures, the body acts as a conductor of electrical activity generated by the heart to the body surface, which can be recorded by body surface electrodes. The various components of the ECG are indicated along with their associated heart function. Parasympathetic regulation of heart rate is solely a negative effect. **Atropine** is the classic cholinergic antagonist ("mAChR blocker"; muscarinic blocker; antimuscarinic). Sympathetic regulation of heart rate is solely a positive effect. **Class II β-blockers** (propanolol, metoprolol, esmolol, sotalol) block β-adrenergic receptors. The antiarrhythmic effect of β-blockers is due to a decrease in phase 4 depolarization in nodal tissue resulting in a decrease SA node activity and AV nodal conduction. The antianginal effect of β-blockers is due to a decrease in heart rate (chronotropism) and a decrease in contractility (inotropism), which decrease myocardial oxygen demand. CN X—cranial nerve X; NE—norepinephrine.

C. **Increases contractility of atrial and ventricular myocytes** by increasing the Ca^{2+} influx associated with phase 2 of the action potential in atrial and ventricular myocytes and increases the activity of the **Ca^{2+} ATPase pump** by **phosphorylation of phospholamban** so that more Ca^{2+} reaccumulates during relaxation and are therefore available for release during later heartbeats. This is also called **positive inotropism.**

XV Electrocardiogram *(Figure 5-7)*

A common way to analyze an electrocardiogram (ECG) is to use the following sequence:

A. **Check voltage calibration.** A 1.0 mV = 10 mm vertical signal is indicated at the beginning or end of a 12-lead ECG. However, in patients with an increased QRS complex, a 1.0 mV = 5 mm vertical signal is used.

B. **Check heart rhythm.** A normal cardiac rhythm is called the **sinus rhythm** and is present when:
   1. Each P wave is followed by a QRS complex.
   2. Each QRS complex is preceded by a P wave.
   3. The P wave is upright in leads I, II, III.
   4. The PR interval is > 0.12 sec.

C. **Calculate heart rate.** There are a number ways to calculate the heart rate from an ECG. Perhaps, the easiest way is to count the number of QRS complexes within 6 seconds and multiply by 10. A normal heart rate = 60–100 beats/min; bradycardia = < 60 beats/min; tachycardia = > 100 beats/min.

D. **Check time intervals.**
   1. Normal PR interval = 0.12–0.20 sec
   2. Normal QRS complex = 0.06–0.10 sec
   3. Normal QT interval = 0.32 sec

E. **Check mean QRS axis.** The normal mean QRS axis is upright in leads I and II (between −30° and +90°).

F. **Check P wave in leads II and V_1.**

G. **Check for QRS complex abnormalities.**

H. **Check for ST-segment and T-wave abnormalities.**

I. **Compare with previous ECGs.**

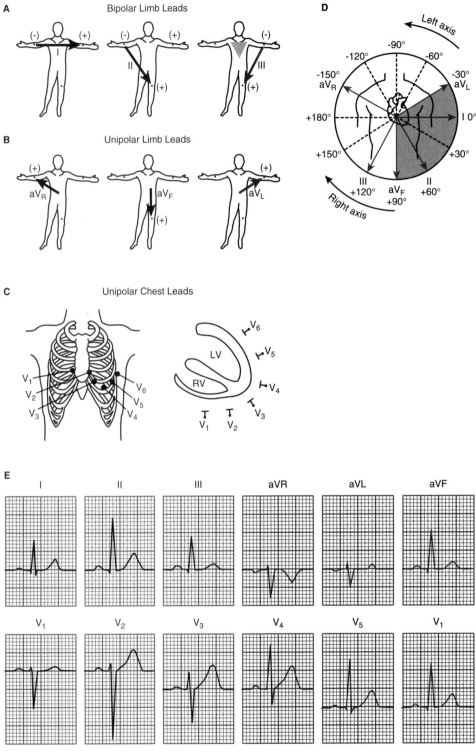

Figure 5-7. **Placement and reading of ECG leads. (A) Three standard bipolar limb leads (I, II, III).** Lead I has electrodes on the right arm and left arm. Lead II has electrodes on the right arm and left leg. Lead III has electrodes on the left arm and left leg. Note the formation of the Einthoven Triangle (*shaded triangle*) by the three bipolar limb leads. **(B) Three augmented unipolar limb leads (aV$_R$, aV$_F$, aV$_L$).** aV$_R$ has an electrode on the right arm. **aV$_F$** has an electrode on the left leg. **aV$_L$** has an electrode on the left arm. **(C) Six precordial unipolar chest leads (V$_1$, V$_2$, V$_3$, V$_4$, V$_5$, V$_6$).** V$_1$ is placed on the right side of the sternum at the 4th intercostal space. V$_2$ is placed on the left side of the sternum at the 4th intercostal space. V$_3$ is placed on the left side between V$_2$ and V$_4$ at the 5th intercostal space. V$_4$ is placed at the 5th intercostal space at the midclavicular line. V$_5$ is placed between V$_4$ and V$_6$ anterior to the axillary line. V$_6$ is placed level with V$_4$ at the midaxillary line. The standard complete ECG prints samples from each of the six limb leads and each of the six chest leads. **(D) Axial reference system is created by overlaying all limb leads.** By convention, limb lead I points to 0°, and measurements of angles proceed clockwise. The normal value for the mean QRS axis is between −30° and +90° (*shaded area*). A mean QRS axis that is more negative than −30° indicates a left-axis deviation. A mean QRS axis that is more positive than +90° indicates a right-axis deviation. **(E) A normal ECG reading from all 12 leads.**

XVI Electrocardiograms of Various Clinical Conditions *(Figure 5-8)*

A Normal Sinus Rhythm
  • Heart rate 60-100/min

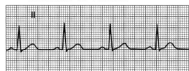

B Sinus Tachycardia
  • Heart rate >100/min

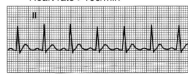

C Sinus Bradycardia
  • Heart rate <60/min

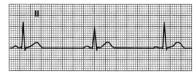

D Atrial Flutter
  • F waves raw-toothed pattern

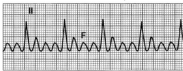

E Atrial Fibrillation
  • *f* waves irregular and weak

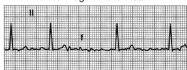

F Premature Ventricular Contraction (PVC)
  • QRS wide and bizarre
  • Complete compensatory pause (*)

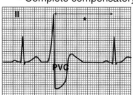

G Ventricular Tachycardia
  • QRS wide, bizarre, identical

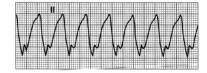

H Ventricular Fibrillation
  • ECG totally erractic
  • Medical emergency

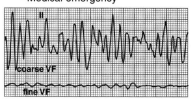

I 1st-Degree Heart Block
  • PR interval > 0.02 sec

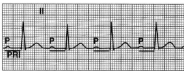

J 2nd-Degree Heart Block (Type I Mobitz)
  • PR interval gradually lengthens
  • P wave but no QRS

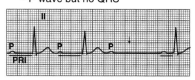

K 3rd-Degree Heart Block (complete)
  • P waves occur independently of QRS

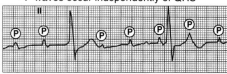

L Right Atrial Hypertrophy
  • P-wave diphasia in V_1
  • Initial deflection > terminal deflection

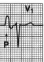

M Left Atrial Hypertrophy
  • P-wave diphasia in V_1
  • Terminal deflection > initial deflection

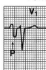

N Right Bundle Block
  • QRS wide and "rabbit ear" pattern
    in V_1 and V_2

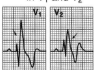

O Left Bundle Block
  • QRS wide and notched in V_5 and V_6

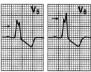

P Right Ventricular Hypertrophy
  • QRS tall and upright in V_1
  • S wave deep in V_6

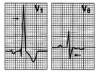

Q Left Ventricular Hypertrophy
  • S wave deep in V_1
  • QRS tall in V_5

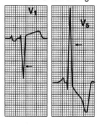

R Early Anterior MI (2-24 h)
  • ST segment elevated in V_3 and V_4

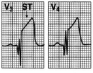

S Recent Anterior MI (24-72 h)
  • Q waves in V_3 and V_4
  • T waves inverted in V_3 and V_4

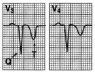

T Old Anterior MI
  • Q waves persist in V_3 and V_4
  • No T-wave inversion

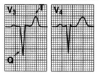

FIGURE 5-8. ECGs of various clinical conditions. (A–K) Heart rhythm and heart rate (arrhythmia) abnormalities. **(L, M)** P-wave abnormalities. **(N–Q)** QRS abnormalities. **(R–T)** ST-segment and T-wave (myocardial infarction) abnormalities

Chapter 6

Pathology

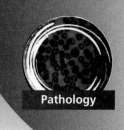

I Atherosclerosis

The characteristic lesion of atherosclerosis is an **atheromatous plaque (fibrofatty plaque; atheroma)** within the **tunica intima** of blood vessels. An early stage in the formation of an atheromatous plaque is the subendothelial **fatty streak.** Fatty streaks are elevated, pale yellow, smooth-surfaced, focal in distribution, and irregular in shape with well-defined borders. An atheromatous plaque may undergo many histological changes to form **complicated plaques.**

A. **Plaque calcification** results in brittle arteries ("brittle pipes").

B. **Plaque hemorrhage** results from tearing of the fibrous cap or rupture of newly formed blood vessels within the plaque.

C. **Plaque rupture** results in **thrombus formation,** whereby the thrombus may partially or completely occlude the lumen (i.e., an **occlusive thrombus**), leading to unstable (crescendo) angina and approximately 90% of all myocardial infarctions (MIs). In this situation, thrombus formation is initiated by platelet aggregation induced by **thromboxane (TXA$_2$).** TXA$_2$ is synthesized from arachidonic acid using the enzyme cyclooxygenase. **Aspirin** covalently inhibits cyclooxygenase, and **nonsteroidal anti-inflammatory drugs (NSAIDs) such as ibuprofen and acetaminophen** reversibly inhibit cyclooxygenase and thereby block the synthesis of TXA$_2$. Consequently, low doses of aspirin and NSAIDs are effective in prevention of MI. Thrombolysis is stimulated by **tissue plasminogen activator (tPA)** treatment, which successfully decreases the extent of ischemic damage due to MI. tPA stimulates the **conversion of plasminogen to plasmin.** Plasmin is a protease that digests fibrin within the thrombus.

II Ischemic Heart Disease

Coronary artery atherosclerosis leads to three major clinical conditions.

A. **Angina pectoris** is the sudden onset of precordial (anterior surface of the body over the heart and stomach) pain. There are three types of angina pectoris:
1. **Prinzmetal (variant) angina** is caused by coronary artery spasms. Attacks occur during rest.
2. **Stable angina** is caused by atherosclerotic narrowing of coronary arteries. Attacks occur during strenuous or excessive activity. This is the most common type of angina.
3. **Unstable (crescendo) angina** is caused by the formation of a thrombus, which occludes the arterial lumen (i.e., occlusive thrombus). MI is imminent.

B. **Myocardial infarction.** An MI is the ischemic necrosis of the myocardium of the heart. **Complications of an MI** include: **hemopericardium** caused by rupture of the free ventricular wall, **arterial emboli, pericarditis** (only in transmural infarcts), and **ventricular aneurysm,** which is a bulge in the heart during systole at the postinfarction scar. **Post-MI syndrome (Dressler's syndrome)** is an autoimmune pericarditis. There are two types of infarcts:

      a. **Transmural infarct** is unifocal and solid and follows the distribution of a specific coronary artery. Pericarditis is common, often causes shock, and is caused by an occlusive thrombus. The volume of **collateral arterial blood flow** is the chief factor that affects the progression of a transmural infarct. In chronic cardiac ischemia, extensive collateral blood vessels develop over time, which supply the subepicardial portion of the myocardium and thereby limit the infarct to the subendocardial portion of the myocardium.

      b. **Subendocardial infarct** is multifocal and patchy and follows a circumferential distribution. Pericarditis is uncommon and is caused by hypoperfusion of the heart (e.g., aortic stenosis, hemorrhagic shock, or hypoperfusion during cardiopulmonary bypass).

C. **Congestive heart failure (CHF).** CHF is the inability of the heart to pump blood at a rate commensurate with the requirements of the body tissues, or the heart can do so only from elevated filling pressures. Most instances of CHF are due to the progressive deterioration of myocardial contractile function (i.e., systolic dysfunction), as occurs in ischemic heart disease or hypertension (i.e., the hypertensive left heart). CHF is characterized by reduced cardiac output (i.e., forward failure) or damming back of blood into the venous system (i.e., backward failure) or both.

III Right Ventricle Failure

A. **General features.** The right ventricle (RV) is susceptible to failure in situations that cause an increase in afterload on the RV. Pure RV failure most often occurs with **cor pulmonale,** which can be induced by intrinsic diseases of the lung or **pulmonary arterial hypertension (PAH). Acute cor pulmonale** is RV dilation caused by a large **thrombopulmonary embolism. Chronic cor pulmonale** is RV hypertrophy followed by RV enlargement and RV failure caused by PAH. PAH is defined as pulmonary artery pressures higher than the normal systolic value of 30 mm Hg. There are **numerous causes of PAH,** which include: **v**asculitis, **i**diopathic (primary PAH), **c**hronic pulmonary emboli, **c**hronic lung disease, **e**mphysema, **E**isenmenger syndrome (mnemonic: VICE)

B. **Clinical findings** include: right hypogastric quadrant discomfort due to hepatomegaly (a cut section of the liver demonstrates a "nutmeg" pattern of chronic passive congestion), peripheral edema (e.g., the hallmark of RV failure is ankle swelling), absent pulmonary edema, jugular vein and portal vein distension, enlarged spleen, peritoneal cavity ascites, pleural effusion, palpable parasternal "heave," S_4 heart sound ("atrial gallop"), and tricuspid valve murmur. Ascent to high altitudes is contraindicated because of hypoxic pulmonary vasoconstriction, which will exacerbate the condition.

IV Left Ventricle Failure

A. **General features.** Left ventricle (LV) failure most often occurs because of impaired LV function caused by MI. The LV is usually hypertrophied and massively dilated. In LV failure, there is progressive damming of blood within the pulmonary circulation such that pulmonary vein pressure mounts and pulmonary edema with wet, heavy lungs is apparent. Coughing is a common feature of LV failure. Transferrin and hemoglobin, which leak from the congested capillaries, are phagocytosed by macrophages in the alveoli (i.e., heart failure cells). In LV failure, the decreased cardiac output causes a reduction in kidney perfusion, which may lead to acute tubular necrosis, and this also activates the renin-angiotensinogen system.

B. **Clinical findings** include: excessive weight; poor diet; episodes of angina; crushing pressure on the chest with pain radiating down the left arm (referred pain); nausea; profuse sweating and cold, clammy skin due to stress-induced release of catecholamines (epinephrine and norepinephrine) from adrenal medulla that stimulate sweat glands and cause peripheral vasoconstriction; dyspnea; orthopnea; auscultation of pulmonary rales due to "popping open" of small airways that were closed off due to pulmonary edema, noisy breathing ("cardiac asthma"); pulmonary wedge pressure (indicator of left atrial pressure) increased versus normal (30 versus 5 mm Hg, respectively); and decreased ejection fraction versus normal (0.35 versus 0.55, respectively).

C. **Treatment** includes: sublingual nitroglycerin; β-adrenergic antagonist (e.g., propanolol β-blocker) to relieve tachycardia and hypertension, although there is a risk because β-blockers further decrease an already compromised cardiac output; intravenous (IV) streptokinase or tPA to reduce the amount of infarcted tissue if administered within 6 hours of MI; atropine to relieve bradycardia; and heparinization and warfarin therapy to prevent ventricular aneurysms, thrombopulmonary embolisms, and deep vein thrombosis.

Ⓥ Cardiomyopathy

Cardiomyopathy is a term used to describe a primary disease of the myocardium. There are three types of cardiomyopathy.

A. **Dilated cardiomyopathy (DCM). DCM is characterized by:** an increased diameter of the four heart chambers (ventricular chambers are more severely affected than atrial chambers) along with a thinning, normal-sized, or thickening of the ventricular wall (or myocardium); a large, flabby heart; myocardial dysfunction **(systolic failure);** cardiac myocyte hypertrophy and atrophy; prominent endocardial and subendocardial fibrosis; and mural thrombi within the LV. DCM is the **most common** type of cardiomyopathy. **The causes of DCM** include: unknown (idiopathic), toxic substances (e.g., alcohol, cobalt, high levels of catecholamines, doxorubicin [Adriamycin], cyclophosphamide, and cocaine), pregnancy, hemochromatosis, and Fabry's disease.

B. **Hypertrophic cardiomyopathy (HCM). HCM is characterized by:** a decreased diameter of the ventricular chambers along with a thickening of the ventricular walls (or myocardium); generally a narrow (slitlike) left ventricular chamber and a massive thickening of the left ventricular wall; asymmetric thickening of the interventricular septum; myocardial dysfunction (**diastolic failure**; i.e., the ventricle cannot fill); prominent papillary muscles and trabeculae carneae; and cardiac myocyte disarray (i.e., oblique and perpendicular arrangement of hypertrophied cardiac myocytes). **The causes of HCM** include: familial with autosomal dominant transmission and mutations in the genes for β-myosin heavy chain, troponin T, α-tropomyosin, and myosin-binding protein C. HCM may be confused with a heart of an athlete.

C. **Restrictive cardiomyopathy (RCM). RCM is characterized by:** a normal diameter of the ventricular chambers along with thickening of the ventricular walls (or myocardium); a primary decrease in ventricular compliance resulting in impaired ventricular filling during diastole (**diastolic failure**) with a relatively normal contractile function of the ventricles; and patchy fibrosis. RCM is the least common type of cardiomyopathy. **The causes of RCM** include: amyloidosis, endomyocardial fibrosis (common in equatorial Africa), Löffler's endocarditis (prominent hypereosinophilia), glycogen storage diseases, and sarcoidosis.

Ⓥ Valvular Heart Disease

A. **Myxomatous degeneration of the mitral valve (mitral valve prolapse; MVP)** is the most common valvular heart disease and most often affects young women. The hallmarks are enlarged, hooded, floppy mitral valve leaflets; prolapse into the left atrium during systole; thrombotic plaques at the leaflet-left atrium border; elongated or ruptured cordae tendineae; dilation of the annulus; concomitant involvement of the tricuspid valve in 20–40% of cases; no commissural fusion (as typically found in rheumatic heart disease). **Clinical findings** include: midsystolic click and a late systolic murmur due to regurgitation.

B. **Calcific aortic stenosis** is common in people over 70 years of age. The hallmark is bulging calcified nodules within the aortic cusps that protrude into the sinuses of Valsalva, which prevent the opening of the cusps. **Clinical findings** include: left ventricular pressure > 200 mm Hg, left ventricular hypertrophy, angina, syncope, and CHF.

C. **Nonbacterial thrombotic endocarditis (marantic endocarditis)** is common in people with a neoplastic condition (e.g., adenocarcinoma or hematological malignancies), disseminated intravascular coagulation syndrome, and wasting non-neoplastic diseases. The hallmark is sterile, noninflammatory vegetations usually on the mitral and aortic valves that grossly resemble infective endocarditis.

D. **Mitral valve calcification** is common in women over 60 years of age, individuals with myxomatous degeneration of the mitral valve, or elevated left ventricular pressures. The hallmark is irregular, stony-hard, occasionally ulcerated calcified nodules within the annulus of the mitral valve behind the leaflets.

Myocarditis

Myocarditis is the generalized inflammation of the myocardium with a prominent interstitial infiltration of T lymphocytes, neutrophils, eosinophils, macrophages, or multinucleate giant cells followed by necrosis of cardiac myocytes and fibrosis in chronic situations. The causes of myocarditis are idiopathic, infectious in origin, or immune related. In the United States, most cases of myocarditis are due to viral infections, particularly **coxsackievirus A** and **B**. Other viruses (e.g., echovirus, influenza virus, human immunodeficiency virus [HIV], and cytomegalovirus) have also been implicated. In South America, most cases of myocarditis are due to protozoan infections, particularly *Trypanosoma cruzi*, which produces **Chagas' disease. Immune-related causes of myocarditis** include: rheumatic fever, rheumatoid arthritis, systemic lupus erythematosus, scleroderma, and hypersensitivity to drugs (e.g., penicillin, sulfonamides, methyldopa, doxorubicin).

Pericarditis

Pericarditis is inflammation of the visceral layer of serous pericardium (known histologically as the epicardium) and the parietal layer of serous pericardium, usually secondary to a variety of cardiac diseases, systemic disorders, or neoplastic metastasis from remote areas. Pericarditis is recognized clinically by a **pericardial friction rub** that results from external compression of the heart.

A. **Types of pericarditis**
   1. **Infectious pericarditis,** caused by viruses or bacteria
   2. **Immune-mediated pericarditis,** caused by rheumatic fever, systemic lupus erythematosus, scleroderma, Dressler's syndrome, or drug hypersensitivity
   3. **Postinfarction pericarditis,** caused by an inflammatory response to necrosis as a result of a transmural infarct
   4. **Postsurgical pericarditis,** caused by opening of the pericardial sac during heart surgery
   5. **Uremic pericarditis,** caused by end-stage renal disease (uremia) probably due to chemical irritation of the pericardium
   6. **Neoplastic pericarditis** (rare), caused by neoplastic metastasis from remote areas

B. Pathological findings in pericarditis

1. **Suppurative pericarditis** presents with a purulent exudate that ranges from thin to creamy pus in which the serosal surfaces are reddened, granular, and coated with the exudate. It is almost always associated with an infectious organism.

2. **Serous pericarditis** presents with a serous or watery exudate (i.e., hydropericardium) in which the serosal surfaces are inflamed with a few neutrophils, lymphocytes, and histiocytes. It is almost always associated with a noninfectious cause.

3. **Serofibrinous pericarditis** presents with a yellow, cloudy, fibrin-rich exudate that contains leukocytes and red blood cells ("bread and butter" pericarditis) in which the serosal surfaces are dry with fine granular roughening.

4. **Fibrosing pericarditis** is a late complication of other forms of pericarditis causing cardiac constriction.

IX Cardiac Tumors

A. **Cardiac myxoma** is the most common primary cardiac tumor (35–50%), most often found in the left atrium. The hallmark is a glistening, gelatinous, 5- to 6-cm mass with a short stalk containing a loose myxoid matrix and stellate-shaped cells. Surgical removal is successful in most cases.

B. **Rhabdomyoma** is the most common primary cardiac tumor in infants and children, most often found in the myocardium of left or right ventricles. The hallmark is multiple, pale, 1-mm to 3-cm nodules containing cells with a central nucleus, abundant glycogen, and fibrillar processes that radiate to the cell margin ("spider cells").

C. **Papillary fibroelastoma** is not a true neoplasm but more appropriately termed a **hamartoma.** The hallmark is 3- to 4-cm papillary fronds growing on the heart valves containing a central dense core of collagen and elastic fibers surrounded by loose connective tissue and covered by endothelium. This hamartoma poses very few clinical problems.

X Selected Photographs, Radiographs, and Micrographs

A. **Coronary artery with atherosclerosis** (*Figure 6-1*)

B. **Myocardial infarction** (*Figure 6-2*)

C. **Right and left ventricle failure** (*Figure 6-3*)

D. **Cardiomyopathy** (*Figure 6-4*)

E. **Valvular heart disease** (*Figure 6-5*)

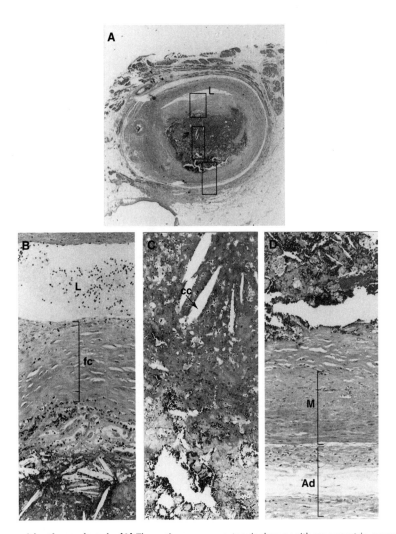

FIGURE 6-1. Coronary artery with atherosclerosis. (A) The entire coronary artery is shown with an eccentric, narrow lumen (*L*) due to the presence of an atheromatous plaque (tunica intima thickening). Atherosclerosis is considered a disease of the **tunica intima. (B–D)** High magnification of the *boxed areas* (shown in **A**) of the **atheromatous plaque.** The fibrous cap (*fc*) is covered by an endothelium and composed of smooth muscle cells, a few macrophages and lymphocytes, and a relatively dense deposition of collagen. The deeper necrotic core (see **C**) consists of a disorganized mass of lipid material, cholesterol crystals (*cc*), cell debris, and foam cells (macrophages digesting modified low-density lipoprotein [LDL]) of the fatty streak. Ad—tunica adventitia; M—tunica media.

▶

FIGURE 6-2. Myocardial infarction (MI). (A) Transmural MIs are caused by thrombotic occlusion of a coronary artery. Infarction is localized to the anatomical area supplied by the occluded artery. Coronary artery occlusion occurs most commonly in the anterior interventricular artery (*AIV;* also called the left anterior descending [*LAD*]), followed by the right coronary artery (*RCA*), and then the left circumflex artery (*LCx*). This is indicated by the numbers 1, 2, and 3. AD—anterior diagonal artery; AM—anterior marginal; IR—intermediate ramus; LMCA—left main coronary artery; OM—obtuse marginal artery; RM—right marginal artery; S—septal branches; SA—sinoatrial artery. **(B)** Serum markers of MI. **Troponin I** is a highly specific cardiac marker that can be detected within 4 hours → 7–10 days after MI pain. **Creatine kinase** (*CK*) consists of M and B subunits. **CK-MM** is found in skeletal muscle and cardiac muscle. CK-MB is found mainly in cardiac muscle. **CK-MB is the test of choice in the first 24 hours after MI pain.** CK-MB begins to rise 4–8 hours after MI pain, peaks at 24 hours, and returns to normal within 48–72 hours. This sequence is important because skeletal muscle injury or non-MI conditions may raise serum CK-MB but do not show this pattern. It is common to calculate the ratio **CK-MB/total CK. A CK-MB/total CK > 2.5%** indicates MI. **Lactate dehydrogenase** (LDH) consists of H and M subunits. LDH-HHHH (*LDH$_1$*) and LDH-HHHM (*LDH$_2$*) are found in cardiac muscle. **LDH$_1$ is the test of choice 2–3 days after MI pain because CK-MB levels have already returned to normal at this time.** It is common to calculate the ratio **DH$_1$/LDH$_2$. An LDH$_1$/LDH$_2$ > 1.0** indicates MI. **(C)** ECGs. An acute MI is associated with ST elevation. A recent MI (within 1–2 days) is associated with deep Q waves and inverted T waves. An old MI (weeks later) is associated with persistence of deep Q waves but no T-wave inversion. **(D)** Evolution of an MI. The histological changes of an MI are indicated.

A

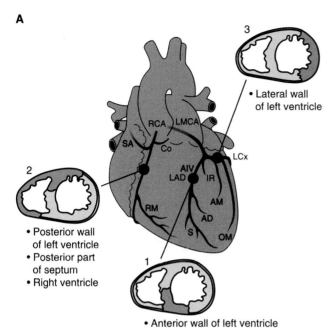

3
• Lateral wall of left ventricle

RCA LMCA
SA
Co
LCx
AIV
LAD IR
RM
AM
S AD
OM

2
• Posterior wall of left ventricle
• Posterior part of septum
• Right ventricle

1
• Anterior wall of left ventricle
• Anterior part of septum

D   Day 1

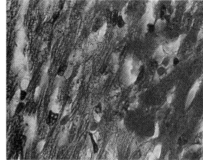

• Coagulation necrosis
• Wavy myocytes
• Pyknotic nuclei
• Eosinophilic cytoplasm
• Contraction bands

B

Troponin I

CK-MB

LDH$_1$

[serum]

1   2

↑
MI pain

Days 2–4

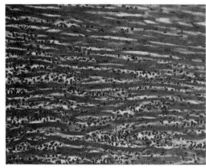

• Total coagulation necrosis
• Loss of nuclei
• Loss of striations
• Dilated vessels (hyperemia)
• Neutrophil infiltration

C Early Anterior MI (2-24 hours)
        • ST segment elevated in V$_3$ and V$_4$

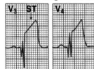

Recent Anterior MI (24-72 hours)
        • Q waves in V$_3$ and V$_4$
        • T waves inverted in V$_3$ and V$_4$

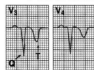

Old Anterior MI
        • Q waves persist in V$_3$ and V$_4$
        • No T-wave inversion

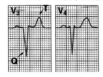

Days 5–10

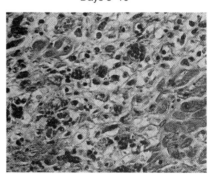

• Macrophage infiltration
• Phagocytosis of necrotic myocytes

Week 7

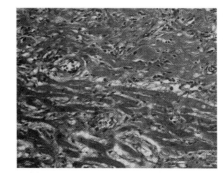

• Collagenous scar

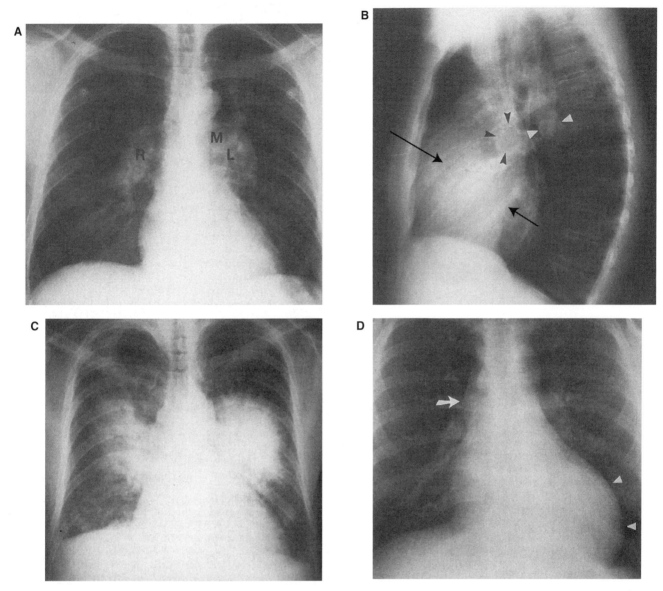

FIGURE 6-3. **(A and B) Right ventricle failure. (A)** Posteroanterior radiograph of pulmonary arterial hypertension (PAH) shows enormously dilated pulmonary trunk (*M*) and right (*R*) and left (*L*) pulmonary arteries with diminutive peripheral pulmonary vessels. **(B)** Lateral radiograph of PAH shows the enlarged right ventricle (RV hypertrophy) and atrium extending anteriorly into the anterior mediastinum (*arrow*). Note that the posterior border of the heart (left ventricle [LV]) is flat (*double arrows*). Fine curvilinear calcifications can be seen outlining the enlarged right and left pulmonary arteries (*arrowheads*). **(C and D) Left ventricle failure. (C)** Anteroposterior (AP) radiograph shows alveolar (air-space) pulmonary edema at the central, parahilar regions of the lung in the classic "bat's wing" appearance. **(D)** AP radiograph shows LV enlargement. Note the prominence of the LV with rounding along the inferior heart border and a downward pointing apex (*arrowheads*).

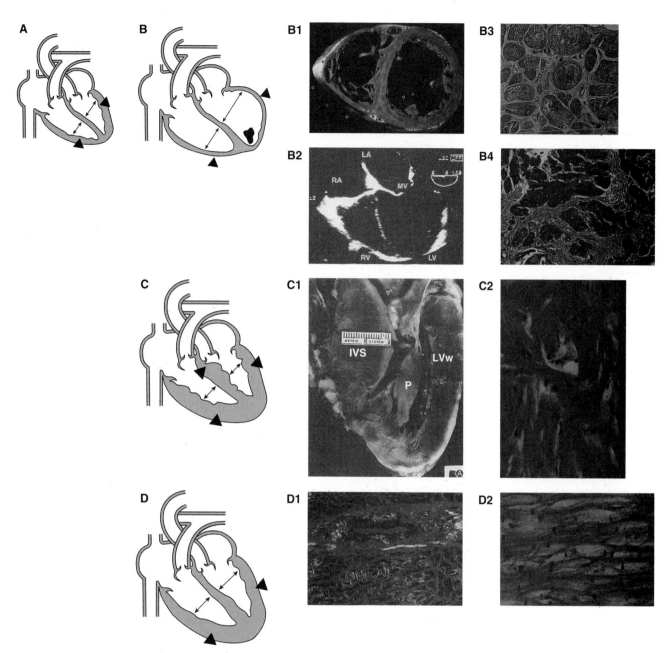

FIGURE 6-4. Cardiomyopathy. (A) Diagram of a normal heart. *Arrows* indicate normal diameter of the ventricular chambers. *Arrowheads* indicate normal-sized ventricular walls. **(B, B1–B4) Dilated cardiomyopathy. (B) Diagram of dilated cardiomyopathy.** *Arrows* indicate the increased diameter of the ventricular chambers. *Arrowheads* indicate an overall thinning of the ventricular walls. Note the mural thrombus in the left ventricle. **(B1)** Photograph of gross specimen of the heart in cross-section shows the increased diameter of the ventricular chambers. Note the thin ventricular wall in some areas. **(B2)** Apical four-chambered echocardiogram shows the increased diameter of the left ventricular chamber. LA—left atrium; LV—left ventricle; MV—mitral valve; RA—right atrium; RV—right ventricle. **(B3)** Light micrograph shows marked cardiac myocyte hypertrophy. **(B4)** Light micrograph shows prominent subendocardial fibrosis surrounding cardiac myocytes. **(C, C1, and C2)** Hypertrophic **cardiomyopathy. (C) Diagram of hypertrophic cardiomyopathy.** *Arrows* indicate the decreased diameter of the ventricular chambers. *Arrowheads* indicate a thickening of the ventricular walls and asymmetrical thickening of the interventricular septum. **(C1)** Photograph of gross specimen of the heart shows thickening for the left ventricular wall (*LVw*) and asymmetrical thickening of the interventricular septum (*IVS*). Note the prominent papillary muscle (*P*). **(C2)** Light micrograph shows oblique and perpendicular arrangement of hypertrophied cardiac myocytes. **(D, D1, and D2) Restrictive cardiomyopathy. (D) Diagram of restrictive cardiomyopathy.** *Arrows* indicate the normal diameter of the ventricular chambers. *Arrowheads* indicate a thickening of the ventricular walls. **(D1)** Light micrograph shows birefringent greenish material (i.e., amyloid) within the intercellular space between cardiac myocytes typically seen in cardiac amyloidosis. Heart tissue was stained with Congo red and photographed under polarizing light. **(D2)** Light micrograph shows an accumulation of glycogen within the cardiac myocytes as typically seen in the glycogen storage disease called Pompe's disease. Cardiac myocytes appear washed out because glycogen is extracted during histological processing.

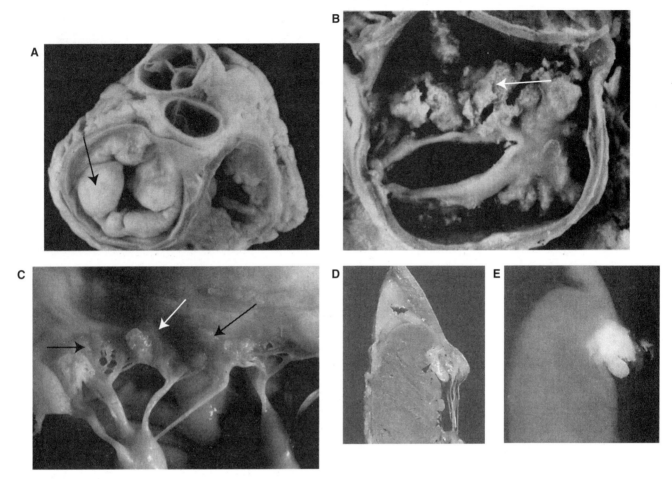

FIGURE 6-5. **Valvular heart disease. (A) Myxomatous degeneration of the mitral valve (mitral valve prolapse).** Photograph of the gross specimen of the heart shows the enlarged, hooded, floppy mitral valve leaflets (*arrow*) protruding into the left atrium. **(B) Calcific aortic stenosis.** Photograph of the gross specimen of the heart shows a congenitally abnormal bicuspid aortic valve. Note the bulging calcified nodules that protrude into the sinus of Valsalva (*arrow*). **(C) Nonbacterial thrombotic endocarditis (marantic endocarditis).** Photograph of the gross specimen of the heart shows the sterile, noninflammatory vegetations (*arrows*) on the normal mitral valve leaflets. **(D and E) Mitral valve calcification. (D)** Photograph of the gross specimen of the heart shows the irregular, stony-hard calcified nodules within the annulus of the mitral valve near the insertion of the posterior mitral valve leaflet. **(E)** Radiograph shows the corresponding area in **D.**

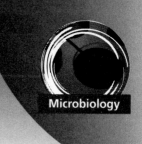

Chapter 7

Microbiology

❶ Rheumatic Carditis (Rheumatic Fever)

A. **General features.** Rheumatic fever (RF) is an immune-mediated inflammation of the heart that occurs in response to streptococcal antigens after an episode of "strep throat" caused by *Streptococcus pyogenes* infection. It occurs principally in children 9 to 11 years of age. RF is a **pancarditis** involving all three layers of the heart. **Pathological findings** include: **verrucous endocarditis,** which consists of sterile, wartlike lesions on the mitral and aortic valves; **myocarditis,** which consists of swollen, eosinophilic collagen surrounded by lymphocytes, plasma cells, and macrophages (called **Aschoff bodies**); **Anitschkow cells,** containing a central band of chromatin that has an "owl-eyed" appearance in cross-section and a "caterpillar" appearance in longitudinal section; and **serofibrinous pericarditis,** which consists of a yellow, cloudy, fibrin-rich exudate that contains leukocytes and red blood cells (RBCs) ("bread and butter" pericarditis), in which the serosal surfaces are dry with fine granular roughening. The clinical diagnosis is made by finding increased antistreptolysin O (ASO) titer in the presence of either two major criteria or one major and two minor criteria based on the Jones criteria. The **major Jones criteria** are polyarthritis, carditis, Sydenham's chorea, erythema induratum, and erythema marginatum. The **minor Jones criteria** are fever, elevated erythrocyte sedimentation rate (ESR), leukocytosis, prolonged PR interval on electrocardiogram (ECG), and history of RF. **Complications** include: **mitral valve stenosis** due to irregular thickening and calcification of the leaflets ("fish mouth" appearance), leading to mitral valve insufficiency and regurgitation (backflow of blood from the left ventricle to the left atrium during systole); **aortic semilunar valve stenosis** due to pronounced thickening of the cusps, leading to aortic valve insufficiency and regurgitation (backflow of blood from the aorta to the left ventricle during diastole); **infective (bacterial) endocarditis** due to bacterial infection of previously scarred heart valve after an episode of bacteremia (e.g., dental procedure); **embolization** due to verrucae detachment and movement to the brain and other organs; and **fibrosing pericarditis.**

B. **Causative agent (*S. pyogenes*; group A).** The genus comprises **gram-positive cocci** that are arranged in pairs or chains, all of which are Gram-positive cocci, facultative anaerobic, and catalase negative. *S. pyogenes* (group A) is a Gram-positive, facultative anaerobe, which is catalase negative, β-hemolytic, and bacitracin-sensitive, and occurs in chains.

C. **Identification.** For pharyngitis: a rapid antigen test is used (if negative, proceed to culture). In a person with repeated positive throat cultures, negative ASO titers suggest a pharyngeal carrier state. For invasive disease: culture is used. For RF: ASO titers > 200 are positive.

D. **Reservoir.** *S. pyogenes* normally colonizes the oropharyngeal mucosa of human carriers.

E. **Virulence factors.** *S. pyogenes* has a **hyaluronic acid capsule** that is resistant to phagocytosis; expresses **M proteins** on the cell surface that convey antigenic variability observed among 80 different serotypes of M proteins; produces **streptolysin O** (oxygen-labile hemolysin), which lyses RBCs, leukocytes, and platelets; produces streptolysin O, which is highly immunogenic; produces antistreptolysin O, which is the basis of the **ASO test;** produces **C5a peptidase,** which degrades C5a that recruits and activates phagocytic cells; produces ***S. pyogenes* erythrogenic toxins (SPE A-C),** which are phage-coded superantigens that activate T cells and macrophages to release cytokines and reduce normal liver clearance of endogenous endotoxin.

F. **Other diseases.** *S. pyogenes* is responsible for other diseases, some of which are much more common clinically.
1. **"Strep throat"** presents as pharyngitis with tonsillar exudate, anterior cervical lymphadenopathy, fever, and nausea.
2. **Scarlatina** (if mild) or **scarlet fever** (if severe) is strep throat with a rash and involves SPE A-C erythrogenic toxins.
3. **Streptococcal impetigo** is characterized by golden-crusted skin lesions.
4. **Necrotizing fasciitis** is the collective effect of *S. pyogenes* virulence factors that cause a rapid, life-threatening infection.
5. **Poststreptococcal sequelae. Acute glomerulonephritis** presents as hypertension, edema, and dark urine due to hematuria or proteinuria. It is usually an M12 serotype and a sequela of pharyngitis or impetigo. **RF fever** presents as fever, carditis, subcutaneous nodules, polyarthritis, and chorea. It is a sequela of untreated *S. pyogenes* pharyngitis.
6. **Streptococcal pneumonia**

Infective (Bacterial) Endocarditis

A. **General features.** Infective endocarditis (IE) is the colonization of heart valves, mural endocardium, or other heart sites most commonly by bacteria (80% of cases are caused by a *Staphylococcus* species) or fungi in immunosuppressed individuals. IE is not caused by viruses. It is a very serious infection characterized by rapidly developing fever, chills, weakness, fatigue, loss of weight, flulike symptoms, and heart murmurs, which may lead to death within days or weeks in 50% of patients despite surgery or antibiotics. **Predisposing factors** include: congenital heart defects (e.g., due to patent ductus arteriosus, tetralogy of Fallot, ventricular septal defects), mitral valve prolapse, rheumatic carditis, intravenous drug use, prosthetic valves, and transient bacteremia (e.g., dental procedure, catheterization, gastrointestinal endoscopy). **Pathological findings** include: large friable vegetations containing thrombotic debris and bacteria usually found on the mitral and aortic semilunar valves and often associated with destruction of underlying cardiac tissues. **Complications** include: congestive heart failure due to valve destruction, embolization due to infected thromboemboli movement to the brain and other organs, glomerulonephritis due to immune-complex deposition (type III hypersensitivity reaction) in the glomeruli ("flea-bitten" kidney), and persistent sepsis.

B. **Causative agents (*viridans* streptococci and *Staphylococcus aureus*).**
1. ***Viridans* streptococci (*e.g., mutans, sanguis*).** The genera are arranged in pairs or chains, all of which are **Gram-positive cocci,** facultative anaerobic, and catalase negative. The *viridans* streptococci are a heterogeneous group of α-hemolytic and nonhemolytic streptococci. *Viridans* streptococci account for most cases of **subacute bacterial endocarditis.** These are not the same bacteria that cause RF.
   a. **Identification.** The *viridans* streptococci are named from the Latin word *viridis* (meaning green), since many of these bacteria produce a green pigment on blood agar medium.
   b. **Reservoir.** The *viridans* streptococci normally colonize the oropharynx, gastrointestinal tract, and genitourinary tract, but are rarely found on the skin surface because fatty acids are toxic to *viridans* streptococci.

c. **Drug resistance.** The *viridans* streptococci have been highly susceptible to penicillin, ampicillin, and most antimicrobial agents in the past. However, moderately resistant and highly resistant *viridans* streptococci have become common in recent years; particularly in the *mitis* group, which includes *S. pneumoniae.* Cephalosporin or vancomycin is used to treat resistant *S. viridans.*

d. **Other diseases.** *S. viridans* infection is responsible for other diseases.

  (1) **Bacteremia** in cancer chemotherapy patients

  (2) **Meningitis** in immunocompromised patients

  (3) **Pneumonia** in immunocompromised patients

  (4) **Dental caries**

2. ***Staphylococcus aureus.*** The genus *Staphylococcus* consists of **Gram-positive cocci** that tend to grow in clusters and are catalase positive. *S. aureus* is Gram positive, aerobic or facultative anaerobic, catalase positive, coagulase positive (initiates the formation of a fibrin clot), β-hemolytic (a clear zone surrounding a bacterial colony grown on blood-agar medium), salt tolerant (haloduric). It contains protein A (binds to Fc fragment of immunoglobulin G [IgG] and inhibits phagocytosis), produces a yellow pigment, and may produce exotoxins. *S. aureus* accounts for most cases of **acute bacterial endocarditis.**

a. **Identification.** *S. aureus* is identified as a Gram-positive *Staphylococcus* that is catalase-positive and coagulase-positive. The screening medium is mannitol-salt medium.

b. **Reservoir.** *S. aureus* normally colonizes the nasopharyngeal mucosa and resides on the skin. It is transmitted by sneezing, skin lesions, and touch with the hands.

c. **Drug resistance.** Methicillin-resistant *Staphylococcus aureus* (MRSA) is due to the acquisition of the ***mecA* gene** that codes for an abnormal **penicillin-binding protein (PBP2′)** that does not bind penicillins. Expression of PBP2′ renders bacteria resistant to all β-lactam antibiotics (including cephalosporins and carbapenems). Most MRSA strains also have plasmid-mediated resistance to other drugs except glycopeptides (e.g., vancomycin).

d. **Virulence factors.** *S. aureus* contains **protein A** on the cell surface that binds the F_c portion of IgG and prevents antibody-mediated clearance of the bacteria. *S. aureus* produces **five cytolytic toxins (α, β, γ, Panton-Valentine leukocidin).** Alpha toxin is a 33,000-d protein that integrates into the host cell membrane (e.g., RBCs, leukocytes, hepatocytes, platelets, and smooth muscle cells) forming 1- to 2-nm pores that lead to osmotic swelling and cell lysis. **Beta toxin (sphingomyelinase C)** is a 35,000-d protein that catalyzes the hydrolysis of phospholipids in the host cell membrane (e.g., RBCs, leukocytes, macrophages, and fibroblasts) proportional to the amount of sphingomyelin exposed on the cell surface. **Delta toxin** is a 3,000-d polypeptide that disrupts the cell membrane and intracellular membranes by a detergent-like action. **Gamma toxin and Panton-Valentine leukocidin** are bicomponent toxins (composed of two polypeptide chains: the S [slow-eluting] component and the F [fast-eluting] component) that integrate into the host cell membrane (e.g., RBCs, neutrophils, macrophages) forming 1- to 2-nm pores that lead to osmotic swelling and cell lysis. *S. aureus* produces **two exfoliative toxins (ETA and ETB). ETA** is a heat-stable serine protease whose gene is chromosomal. **ETB** is a heat-labile serine protease and is plasmid-mediated. ETA and ETB promote the splitting of desmosomes within the stratum granulosum of the skin epidermis. *S. aureus* produces **eight enterotoxins (A-E, G-I).** All the enterotoxins are heat stable (heating to 100°C for 30 minutes) and hydrolysis resistant to gastric and jejunal enzymes. The precise mechanism of action is not known; however, these enterotoxins are superantigens that activate T cells, causing release of cytokines and mast cells that cause release of inflammatory mediators.

S. aureus produces **toxic shock syndrome toxin-1 (TSST-1).** TSST-1 is a 22,000-d heat-stable, proteolysis-resistant protein whose gene is chromosomal. TSST-1 is a superantigen that activates T cells and macrophages, causing release of cytokines, and reduces normal liver clearance of endogenous endotoxin.

  e. Other diseases. *S. aureus* is responsible for causing other diseases, some of which are much more common clinically.

    (1) *S. aureus* **food poisoning** presents as rapid onset (1–6 hours) of abdominal pain, vomiting, and diarrhea caused by heat-stable enterotoxins (A–E, G–I) produced in poorly refrigerated *S. aureus*–contaminated foods.

    (2) *S. aureus* **skin or subcutaneous infections** present as subcutaneous tenderness and heat, redness, and swelling with a surgery or neutropenia predisposition. This infection may lead to **scalded skin syndrome** if exfoliative toxins ETA and ETB are produced. **Staphylococcal impetigo** is characterized by large bullae (vesicles).

    (3) Toxic shock syndrome (TSS) presents as fever, hypotension, scarlatiniform rash, desquamation of palms and soles, multiorgan failure with surgical packing or super tampon use predisposition. TSST-1 plays a prominent role.

    (4) Staphylococcal pneumonia.

Myocarditis

Myocarditis is the generalized inflammation of the myocardium with a prominent interstitial infiltration of T lymphocytes, neutrophils, eosinophils, macrophages, or multinucleate giant cells followed by necrosis of cardiac myocytes and fibrosis in chronic situations. The causes of myocarditis may be idiopathic, infectious, or immune related.

A. Viral myocarditis

  1. Causative agent (coxsackievirus B). Coxsackie B, belonging to the **Picornaviridae virus family,** is a **nonsegmented, single-stranded, positive sense RNA (ss + RNA) virus.** The virion is a **naked** (nonenveloped) 30-nm **iscosahedron.** The Picornaviridae family is divided into two main genera: the *Enterovirus* **genus** (which includes poliovirus, coxsackievirus, echovirus, enteroviruses 68–71, and hepatitis A—all acid stable) and the *Rhinovirus* **genus** (which consists of at least 100 serotypes of rhinoviruses—all acid labile). Coxsackie B virus has tightly fitting capsomers consisting of four virion proteins **(VP0, VP1–VP4),** which are involved in binding to the host cell. The coxsackie B virus genome has a 3′ poly A tail that enhances infectivity and a 5′ **VP$_g$ protein** that plays a role in viral RNA packaging into the capsid and initiating viral RNA synthesis. The coxsackie B virus genome encodes for the capsomers (VP0, VP1–VP4), VP$_g$, at least two proteases, and RNA-dependent RNA polymerase. Coxsackie B is insensitive to acid pH and is difficult to inactivate with disinfectants or organic solvents.

  2. Replication

  a. Infection and entry. The coxsackie B virus infects the host cell through **VP1** capsomer protein binding to host cell intercellular adhesion molecule **1 (ICAM-1)** or some other receptor specific for cardiac myocytes. Upon binding, VP4 is released and the viral genome is injected directly across the host cell membrane (called **viropexis**).

  b. Early transcriptional events. The viral +RNA is used as mRNA and is translated within the cytoplasm into one large polypeptide, which is cleaved into various viral proteins.

  c. Replication of viral genome. Viral +RNA replication occurs in the host cell cytoplasm and is mediated by RNA-dependent RNA polymerase. The viral +RNA is first transcribed into a −RNA template, which then undergoes replication to the viral +RNA genome. VP$_g$ is attached to the 5′ end.

d. **Viral assembly.** The viral proteins (VP0, VP1–VP4) associate to form the capsid, and the viral +RNA genome is inserted inside the capsid.

e. **Viral release.** The virion is released by cell lysis.

3. **Identification.** Coxsackievirus B can be grown on primary monkey or human embryo kidney cells. The specific type of enterovirus can be determined by specific antibody and antigen assays or reverse transcriptase polymerase chain reaction (RT-PCR) to detect specific viral RNA. Coxsackieviruses can usually be isolated from the throat, stool, and cerebrospinal fluid (meningitis) during infection. However, coxsackie B virus is rarely isolated in patients with myocarditis because the symptoms occur several weeks after infection. Coxsackieviruses are named for the town in Coxsackie, New York, where the virus was first isolated. The coxsackieviruses are divided into group A and group B (body) based on certain biological and antigenic differences.

4. **Reservoir.** Coxsackievirus B has a tropism to infect cardiac myocytes within the myocardium of the heart. Enterovirus outbreaks occur mainly in the summer and spread readily in schools and day care centers. Enteroviruses are transmitted by the fecal–oral route, which is fostered by poor sanitation, crowded living conditions, and sewage contamination of drinking water. They are exclusively human pathogens and, contrary to their name, do not cause enteric diseases. Rather, the disease is determined by differences in viral tropism to various receptor-bearing target tissues and cytolytic capacity of the virus.

B. Parasitic myocarditis

1. **General features.** *Trypanosoma cruzi* causes Chagas' disease in humans. The earliest signs of Chagas' disease is a chagoma (erythematous, indurated area) followed by a rash and edema around the eyes and face. **Clinical signs of acute infection** include: fever, chills, malaise, myalgia, and fatigue. **Clinical signs of chronic infection** include: myocarditis, hepatosplenomegaly, and enlargement of the esophagus and colon due to destruction of neurons (e.g., myenteric plexus).

2. **Causative agent (*Trypanosoma cruzi*).** *T. cruzi* is a flagellated protozoan, which is a single-celled parasite.

3. **Life cycle**

a. **Infection and entry.** *T. cruzi* infects humans when a reduviid bug (kissing bug) bites a person (usually in the facial area), feeds on blood and tissue fluid, and then defecates into the bite wound. The **trypomastigote is the infective stage of *T. cruzi*** and has a flagellum; a full-length undulating membrane is present in the feces and enters the bite wound.

b. **Human host events.** The trypomastigote enters the blood and penetrates various human tissues (cardiac myocytes, liver, brain). Within the tissues, the trypomastigote loses its flagellum and undulating membrane to develop into a small, oval-shaped **amastigote (the intracellular stage of *T. cruzi*).** The amastigote divides by binary fission, enters new host cells, destroys host cells to become liberated, and enters the blood to revert back to the trypomastigote stage.

c. **Reduviid bug events.** A reduviid bug bites an infected human and ingests trypomastigotes that are present in the human blood. The ingested trypomastigotes travel to the midgut of the reduviid bug and develop into **epimastigotes.** The epimastigotes divide by binary fission, travel to the hindgut, and develop into trypomastigotes, which are present in the reduviid bug feces ready to initiate a new human infection.

4. **Identification.** *T. cruzi* (trypomastigotes) can be identified in blood films or anticoagulated blood early in the infection. *T. cruzi* (amastigotes) can be identified in tissue biopsies (lymph node, spleen, liver,) later in the infection.

5. **Reservoir.** *T. cruzi* is found in reduviid bugs in North, Central, and South America. Chagas' disease is found most often in children of Central and South America and is rare in the United States.

Ⅳ Selected Photographs, Radiographs, and Micrographs

A. Rheumatic carditis (rheumatic fever) *(Figure 7-1)*

B. Infective (bacterial) endocarditis *(Figure 7-2)*

C. Viral and parasitic myocarditis *(Figure 7-3)*

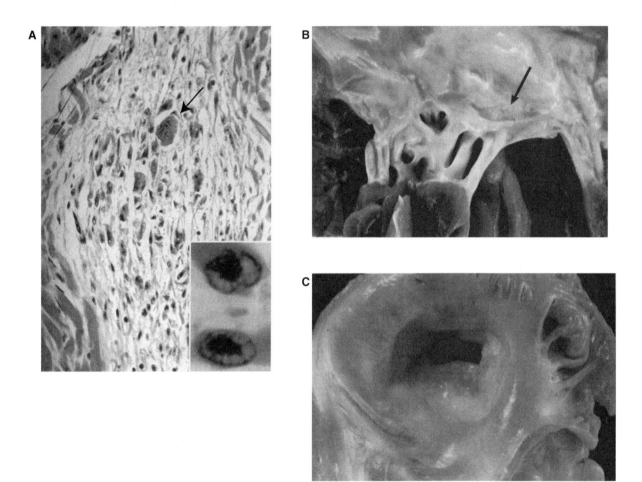

FIGURE 7-1. Rheumatic carditis (rheumatic fever). (A) Light micrograph shows an Aschoff body within the myocardium consisting of degenerating collagen, a multinucleated giant cell (Aschoff myocyte; *arrow*), and lymphocytes. The *inset* shows Anitschkow myocyte nuclei with an owl-eyed appearance in cross-section and a caterpillar appearance in longitudinal section. **(B)** Photograph of gross specimen shows a thickened, focally calcified (*arrow*) mitral valve leaflet and short, thick, and fused chordae tendineae. **(C)** Photograph of gross specimen (viewed from the left atrium) shows a thickened, rigid mitral valve with fused leaflets, creating a narrow orifice ("fish-mouth" appearance) characteristic of rheumatic mitral valve stenosis.

▶

FIGURE 7-3. (A and B) Viral myocarditis. (A) Diagram of coxsackievirus B replication. ICAM-1—intercellular adhesion molecule-1. **(B)** Light micrograph shows prominent interstitial infiltration of T lymphocytes, neutrophils, eosinophils, and macrophages within the myocardium of the heart. **(C and D) Parasitic myocarditis. (C)** Diagram of the life cycle of *Trypanosoma cruzi.* (D) Light micrograph shows the small, oval-shaped amastigotes (intracellular stage of *T. cruzi*) within the myocardium of the heart.

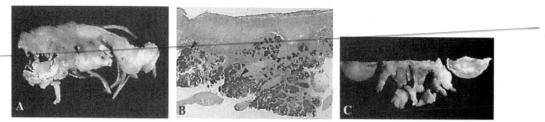

FIGURE 7-2. Infective (bacterial) endocarditis. (A) Photograph of gross specimen shows an excised mitral valve with prolapse, ruptured chordae tendineae, and bulky vegetations (*arrowheads*) that partially destroyed the valve leaflet. This excised mitral valve is from a 52-year-old man who underwent valve replacement and had mitral valve regurgitation, low-grade fever, and a mitral valve vegetation revealed by echocardiography. **(B)** Light micrograph of the excised mitral valve in **A** shows vegetation on the valve surface, which consists of fibrin-containing bacterial colonies (*arrowheads*) and interspersed inflammatory cells. **(C)** Photograph of gross specimen shows an excised aortic valve with a large vegetation on the middle aortic valve cusp, which resulted in multiple perforations. This excised aortic valve is from a 35-year-old intravenous drug abuser with acute aortic regurgitation and congestive heart failure.

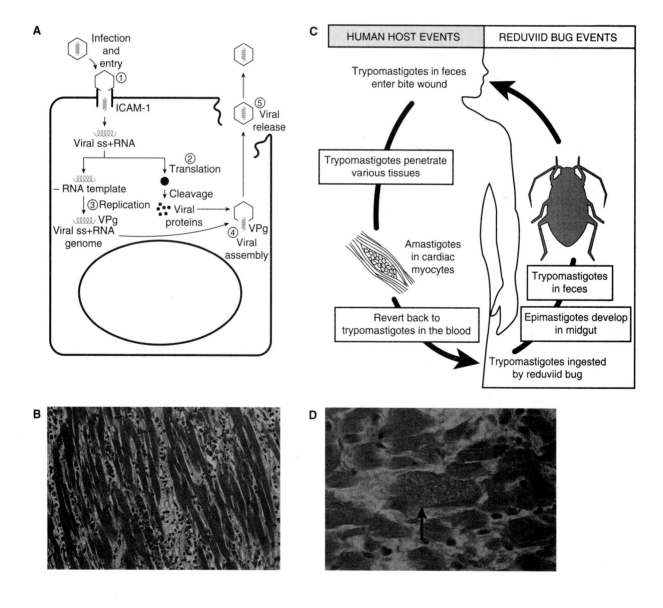

Chapter 8

Pharmacology

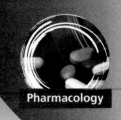

❶ Definitions

A. Excitability is the capacity of a cell to generate an action potential in the presence of an external depolarizing stimulus.

B. Automaticity is the capacity of a cell to generate a depolarization in the absence of an external depolarizing stimulus.

C. Effective refractory period (ERP) refers to a short time past the absolute refractory period during which a cardiac myocyte produces a localized action potential that does not propagate in response to a new stimulus.

❷ Antiarrhythmic Drugs (Table 8-1; Figure 8-1)

A. Class IA drugs

1. **Quinidine (Quinaglute, Quinidex)** is a **fast Na⁺ ion channel antagonist** that binds to open Na⁺ channels and blocks Na⁺ influx. This results in: **decreased excitability and conduction velocity** due to reducing the slope of the phase 0 depolarization and amplitude of the action potential; **decreased automaticity** due to reducing the slope of the phase 4 depolarization shifting the threshold voltage upward towards zero; **increased ERP** due to the long duration of the action potential; ↑ QRS interval; and ↑ QT interval. Quinidine is also an **M₂ muscarinic acetylcholine receptor (M₂AChR) antagonist** that acts at the sinoatrial (SA) and atrioventricular (AV) nodes, which are main sites of parasympathetic innervation. **Clinical uses** include: atrial flutter, atrial fibrillation, ventricular arrhythmias, and supraventricular arrhythmias. Quinidine may cause a **lupus-like syndrome** with symptoms including: polyarthritis, fever, and pleuritic chest pain. **Quinidine syncope** is associated with: long QT interval, lightheadedness, fainting, and an oscillatory cardiac rhythm called **torsades de pointes,** which is potentially lethal. **Quinidine toxicity (cinchonism)** has the following symptoms: headache, dizziness, and tinnitus.

2. **Procainamide (Procan-SR, Pronestyl)** is similar to quinidine but is not an **M₂AChR antagonist.**

3. **Disopyramide (Norpace)** is similar to quinidine but is a more potent **M₂AChR antagonist** and has the longest half-life of all class I drugs.

B. Class IB drugs

1. **Lidocaine (Xylocaine)** is a **fast Na⁺ channel antagonist** that binds to open or closed Na⁺ channels (greater effect on closed Na⁺ channels) and blocks Na⁺ influx. This results in: **decreased excitability and conduction velocity** due to reducing the slope of the phase 0 depolarization and amplitude of the action potential; **decreased automaticity** due to reducing the slope of the phase 4 depolarization, shifting the threshold voltage upward toward zero; and **decreased ERP** due to the short duration of the action potential (unexpected action). Lidocaine is not an M₂AChR antagonist. Lidocaine is administered intravenously and has a half-life of 20 minutes. **Clinical uses** include: ventricular tachycardia, premature ventricular

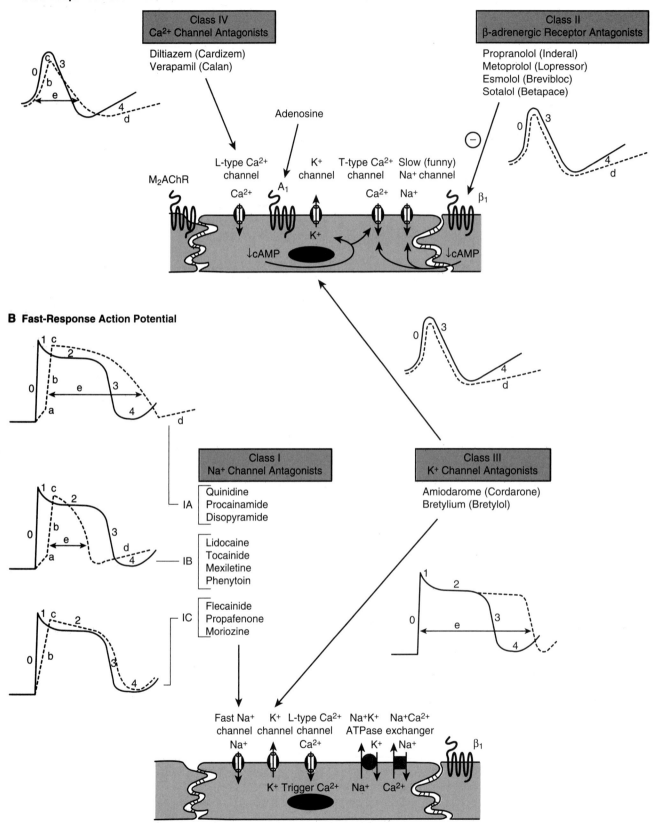

A Slow-Response Action Potential

Class IV
Ca²⁺ Channel Antagonists

Diltiazem (Cardizem)
Verapamil (Calan)

Adenosine

Class II
β-adrenergic Receptor Antagonists

Propranolol (Inderal)
Metoprolol (Lopressor)
Esmolol (Brevibloc)
Sotalol (Betapace)

M₂AChR

L-type Ca²⁺
channel

K⁺
channel

T-type Ca²⁺
channel

Slow (funny)
Na⁺ channel

β₁

B Fast-Response Action Potential

Class I
Na⁺ Channel Antagonists

Quinidine
Procainamide
Disopyramide   IA

Lidocaine
Tocainide
Mexiletine
Phenytoin   IB

Flecainide
Propafenone
Moriozine   IC

Class III
K⁺ Channel Antagonists

Amiodarome (Cordarone)
Bretylium (Bretylol)

Fast Na⁺
channel

K⁺
channel

L-type Ca²⁺
channel

Na⁺K⁺
ATPase

Na⁺Ca²⁺
exchanger

β₁

FIGURE 8-1. Diagram of antiarrhythmic drug action. (A) Slow-response action potential found in the SA node and AV node. A₁—A₁ adenosine receptor; β₁—β₁-adrenergic receptor; M₂AChR—M₂ muscarinic acetylcholine receptor. **(B)** Fast-response action potential found in atrial myocytes, bundle of His, Purkinje myocytes, and ventricular myocytes. The effect of the various drugs on the action potential curves is shown. *Solid line*—normal action potential; *dotted line*—drug; 0, 1, 2, 3, 4—phases of the normal action potential; a—threshold; b—phase 0; slope c—amplitude of action potential; d—phase 4; slope e—effective refractory period.

complexes, ventricular fibrillation, and digitalis-induced ventricular arrhythmia. **Lidocaine toxicity** has the following symptoms: drowsiness, vertigo, twitching, and disorientation, and, at high plasma concentrations (< 9 μg/mL), psychosis, convulsions, and respiratory depression.

2. **Tocainide (Tonocard)** is similar to lidocaine and is administered PO (by mouth).

3. **Mexiletine (Mexitil)** is similar to lidocaine, is administered PO, and has a long half-life.

4. **Phenytoin (Dilantin)** is an anticonvulsant drug and an Na^+ channel antagonist that binds to closed Na^+ channels and blocks Na^+ influx.

C. Class IC drugs

1. **Flecainide (Tambocor) is a fast Na^+ channel antagonist** that binds to Na^+ channels and blocks Na^+ influx. This results in: **decreased excitability and conduction velocity** due to reducing the slope of the phase 0 depolarization and amplitude of the action potential; **normal automaticity,** since there is no effect on the phase 4 depolarization; **normal ERP,** since there is no effect on the duration of the action potential; $\uparrow$ QRS interval; $\uparrow$ QT interval; and $\uparrow$ PR interval. Flecainide is administered PO. **Clinical uses** include: ventricular arrhythmias and supraventricular arrhythmias in patients without structural heart damage.

2. **Propafenone (Rythmol)** is similar to flecainide and is also a β-adrenergic receptor antagonist.

3. **Moricizine (Ethmozine)** is similar to flecainide and is also an **M_2AChR antagonist.**

D. Class II drugs

1. **Propranolol (Inderal) is a nonselective $β_1$- and $β_2$-adrenergic receptor antagonist** that blocks the effects of the sympathetic nervous system on the heart. Remember that postganglionic sympathetic axons innervating the heart release norepinephrine (NE). NE binds to the $β_1$-adrenergic receptor, which is a **G_s-protein–linked receptor** that stimulates the adenylate cyclase and increases cyclic adenosine 3′, 5′ monophosphate (cAMP) levels. A β-adrenergic receptor antagonist decreases cAMP levels. This results in the following antiarrhythmic effects: **decreased automaticity of the SA node** (and **ectopic pacemakers**) and **decreased conduction velocity of the AV node** owing to reducing the slope of the phase 4 depolarization most likely caused by deactivation of the **T-type Ca^{2+} channel** and the **slow (funny) Na^+ channel.** Clinical uses include: supraventricular arrhythmias, ventricular tachycardia, and digitalis-induced arrhythmia. Propranolol is also used to treat angina and hypertension, which is discussed under IV. Antianginal Drugs and V. Antihypertensive Drugs.

2. **Metoprolol (Lopressor)** is a cardioselective **$β_1$-adrenergic receptor antagonist** and has antiarrhythmic effects similar to those of propranolol.

3. **Esmolol (Brevibloc)** is a **cardioselective $β_1$-adrenergic receptor antagonist** and has antiarrhythmic effects similar to those of propranolol.

4. **Sotalol (Betapace)** is a nonselective **$β_1$ and $β_2$-adrenergic receptor antagonist** and has antiarrhythmic effects similar to those of propranolol. Sotalol is also a **K^+ channel antagonist.**

E. Class III drugs

1. **Amiodarone (Cordarone)** is a **K^+ channel antagonist** that binds to K^+ channels and blocks K^+ efflux. This results in: **increased ERP in atrial myocytes, bundle of His, Purkinje myocytes, and ventricular myocytes** due to the long duration of the action potential; **decreased automaticity of the SA node and AV nodes** due to reducing the slope of the phase 4 depolarization. Amiodarone is a **thyroid hormone analogue (T_3 and T_4)** and an **α-adrenergic receptor antagonist** (which causes coronary and peripheral vasodilation). Amiodarone has a very long half-life of 100 days. **Clinical uses** include: ventricular arrhythmias and supraventricular arrhythmias.

2. **Bretylium (Bretylol)** is similar to amiodarone.

F. **Class IV drugs**
1. **Diltiazem (Cardizem)** is an **L-type Ca^{2+} channel antagonist** that binds to Ca^+ channels and blocks Ca^+ influx. This results in the following antiarrhythmic effects: **decreased excitability of the SA node and decreased conduction velocity of the AV node** due to reducing the slope of the phase 0 depolarization and amplitude of the action potential; **decreased automaticity** due to reducing the slope of the phase 4 depolarization; and **increased ERP** due to the long duration of the action potential. **Clinical uses** include: supraventricular arrhythmias. Diltiazem is also used to treat angina and hypertension.
2. **Verapamil (Calan, Isoptin, Verelan)** is similar to diltiazem.

G. **Adenosine (Adenocard) is a A_1-receptor agonist.** Adenosine binds to the A-receptor, which is a G_1-protein–linked receptor that inhibits adenylate cyclase and decreases cAMP levels. This results in: **decreased automaticity, short duration of the action potential,** and **hyperpolarization in the SA and AV nodes** due to activation of the K^+ channels (raises K^+ efflux); **increased refractory nature of the AV node** due to deactivation of the T-type Ca^{2+} channels. Adenosine has an extremely short half-life of 10 seconds and is administered intravenously. **Clinical uses** include: supraventricular arrhythmias (drug of choice for acute termination).

Ⅲ Congestive Heart Failure Drugs *(Figure 8-2)*

A. **Direct vasodilators**
1. **Hydralazine (Apresoline)** is an **arteriolar vasodilator** that acts directly on vascular smooth muscle (mechanism unknown). This results in: **decreased peripheral vascular resistance (PVR).** **Clinical uses** include: congestive heart failure (CHF) and hypertension.
2. **Minoxidil (Loniten;** a prodrug metabolized to minoxidil sulfate) is a **K^+ channel agonist** that activates K^+ channels and raises K^+ efflux. Minoxidil is an **arteriolar vasodilator** that acts directly on vascular smooth muscle. This results in: **decreased PVR** due to hyperpolarization and relaxation of arteriolar smooth muscle. **Clinical uses** include: CHF and hypertension.
3. **Sodium nitroprusside (Nitropress;** metabolized to **nitric oxide [NO]** in vascular smooth muscle). NO is **a guanylate cyclase activator** that raises the level of guanosine 3′, 5′ cyclic monophosphate (cGMP) in vascular smooth muscle. Guanylate cyclase catalyzes the conversion of guanosine 5′-triphosphate (GTP) → cGMP, which inhibits Ca^{2+} binding and dephosphorylates the myosin light chain. This leads to vascular smooth muscle relaxation. Sodium nitroprusside is an **arteriolar and venous vasodilator.** This results in: **decreased PVR** due to relaxation of arteriolar and venous smooth muscle; **decreased preload** (load on the ventricular myocytes at the end of diastole); and **decreased afterload** (load on the ventricular myocytes during systole). **Clinical uses** include: CHF and hypertensive emergencies.

B. **Phosphodiesterase (PDE) inhibitors. Amrinone (Inocor) and milrinone (Primacor)** are **cAMP phosphodiesterase inhibitors** that raise the level of cAMP in cardiac muscle and vascular smooth muscle. cAMP phosphodiesterase catalyzes the conversion of camp → adenosine 5′-triphosphate (ATP). This results in: **increased contractility of**

▶

FIGURE 8-2. Diagram of congestive heart failure drug action. (A) Vascular smooth muscle. α_1—α_1-adrenergic receptor; ATP—adenosine 5′-triphosphate; β_2—β_2-adrenergic receptor; NO—nitric oxide; PVR—peripheral vascular resistance. **(B)** SA and AV node (slow-response action potential). A_1—A_1 adenosine receptor; M_2AChR—M_2 muscarinic acetylcholine receptor. **(C)** Atrial and ventricular myocytes (fast-response action potential). β_1—β_1-adrenergic receptor; PDE—phosphodiesterase. **(D)** Lung capillaries. The endothelium of lung capillaries are the major site of angiotensin I → angiotensin II conversion. **(E)** Kidney. ATL—ascending thin limb of the loop of Henle; BC—Bowman's capsule; CD—collecting ducts; DCT—distal convoluted tubule; DST—distal straight tubule; DTL—descending thin limb of the loop of Henle; PCT—proximal convoluted tubule.

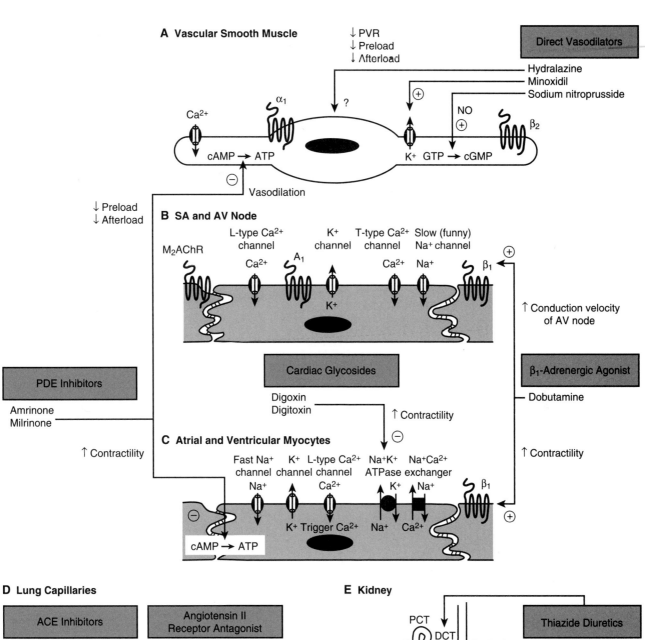

A Vascular Smooth Muscle

↓ PVR
↓ Preload
↓ Afterload

Direct Vasodilators

Hydralazine
Minoxidil
Sodium nitroprusside

Ca^{2+} α_1 ?   ⊕   NO ⊕ β_2

cAMP → ATP   ⊖ K^+ GTP → cGMP

Vasodilation

↓ Preload
↓ Afterload

B SA and AV Node

M_2AChR L-type Ca^{2+} channel K^+ channel   T-type Ca^{2+} channel   Slow (funny) Na^+ channel   ⊕

Ca^{2+} A_1 Ca^{2+} Na^+ β_1

K^+

↑ Conduction velocity of AV node

Cardiac Glycosides

PDE Inhibitors

Amrinone
Milrinone

Digoxin
Digitoxin

↑ Contractility

⊖

β_1-Adrenergic Agonist

Dobutamine

↑ Contractility

↑ Contractility

C Atrial and Ventricular Myocytes

Fast Na^+ channel K^+ channel   L-type Ca^{2+} channel Na^+K^+ ATPase Na^+Ca^{2+} exchanger β_1

Na^+ Ca^{2+} K^+ Na^+

⊖

K^+ Trigger Ca^{2+} Na^+ Ca^{2+} ⊕

cAMP → ATP

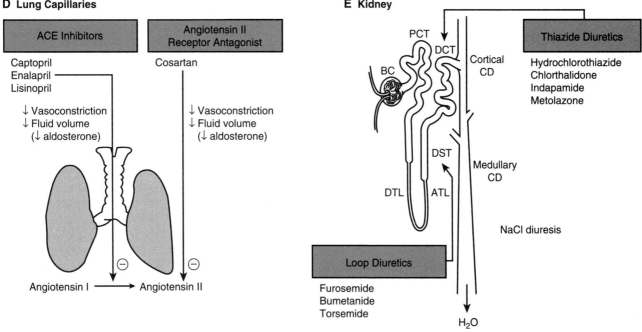

D Lung Capillaries

ACE Inhibitors

Captopril
Enalapril
Lisinopril

↓ Vasoconstriction
↓ Fluid volume
(↓ aldosterone)

Angiotensin II Receptor Antagonist

Cosartan

↓ Vasoconstriction
↓ Fluid volume
(↓ aldosterone)

⊖   ⊖

Angiotensin I → Angiotensin II

E Kidney

PCT   DCT   Cortical CD

Thiazide Diuretics

Hydrochlorothiazide
Chlorthalidone
Indapamide
Metolazone

BC

DST   Medullary CD

DTL   ATL

NaCl diuresis

Loop Diuretics

Furosemide
Bumetanide
Torsemide

H_2O

atrial and ventricular myocytes (or positive inotropism), decreased preload, and decreased afterload due to the vasodilation.

C. **Cardiac glycosides. Digoxin (Lanoxin) and digitoxin (Crystodigin) are Na$^+$-K$^+$ ATPase inhibitors** that elevate intracellular Na$^+$ ions. The elevated Na$^+$ ions overwhelm the Na$^+$-Ca^{2+} exchanger so that more Ca^{2+} ions can be reaccumulated by the terminal cisternae (TCs). During the next contraction, more Ca^{2+} ions are released from the TCs increasing the force of contraction. This results in: **increased contractility of atrial and ventricular myocytes (or positive inotropism).** The antiarrhythmic effect of cardiac glycosides is due to their indirect effect on the autonomic nervous system (increase parasympathetic activity and decrease sympathetic activity). **Clinical uses** include: CHF, atrial flutter, and atrial fibrillation. **Side effects** include: nausea, vomiting, and diarrhea.

D. **β-Adrenergic agonist. Dobutamine (Dobutrex) is a β-adrenergic agonist** that activates β$_1$-adrenergic receptors (raises the level of cAMP) and raises the sympathetic activity of the heart. This results in: **increased contractility of atrial and ventricular myocytes (or positive inotropism)** and **increased conduction velocity of the AV node (or positive dromotropism). Clinical uses** include: CHF and shock.

E. **Angiotensin-converting enzyme (ACE) inhibitors. Captopril (Capoten), enalapril (Vasotec), and lisinopril (Prinivil) are ACE inhibitors** that reversibly inhibit ACE and prevent the conversion of angiotensin I → angiotensin II (a potent vasoconstrictor), leading to low levels of angiotensin II. This results in: **decreased vasoconstriction** due to the low levels of angiotensin II and **decreased fluid volume** due to low levels of aldosterone (caused by low levels of angiotensin II). **Clinical uses** include: CHF and hypertension.

F. **Angiotensin II receptor antagonist. Losartan (Cozaar;** metabolized to more potent 5-carboxylic acid form) is an **angiotensin II receptor antagonist** that blocks the action of angiotensin II (a potent vasoconstrictor). This results in: **decreased vasoconstriction** due to the blocked action of angiotensin II and **decreased fluid volume** due to low levels of aldosterone (caused by the blocked action of angiotensin II). **Clinical use** includes: hypertension.

G. **Diuretics**
   1. **Loop diuretics (sulfonamide derivatives). Furosemide (Lasix; "lasts six" hours), bumetanide (Bumex), and torsemide (Demadex) are Na$^+$-K$^+$-2Cl$^-$-symporter inhibitors** that act on the **distal straight tubule (DST) of the loop of Henle** and cause a decreased NaCl reabsorption (tubular fluid → plasma). This results in: **NaCl diuresis; hypokalemic alkalosis** due to the delivery of large amounts of Na$^+$ to the cortical collecting duct causing K$^+$ secretion (blood → tubular fluid ; K$^+$ wasting) and H$^+$ secretion (plasma → tubular fluid). **Clinical uses** include: edema associated with CHF, liver disease, renal disease, pulmonary disease, and hypertension (due to decrease in blood volume).
   2. **Thiazide diuretics (sulfonamide derivatives). Hydrochlorothiazide (HydroDIURIL), chlorthalidone (Hygroton), indapamide (Lozol), and metolazone (Mykrox) are Na$^+$-Cl$^-$ symporter inhibitors** that act on the early **distal convoluted tubule (DCT)** and cause a decreased NaCl reabsorption (tubular fluid → plasma). This results in: **NaCl diuresis; hypokalemic alkalosis** due to the delivery of large amounts of Na$^+$ to the cortical collecting duct causing K$^+$ secretion (plasma → tubular fluid; K$^+$ wasting) and H$^+$ secretion (plasma → tubular fluid). **Clinical uses** include: edema associated with CHF, liver disease, renal disease, and corticosteroid therapy; hypertension (due to decrease in blood volume).

Ⅳ Antianginal Drugs *(Table 8-1; Figure 8-3)*

A. **Nitrates. (Nitroglycerin [Nitrostat], isosorbide dinitrate [Isordil], amyl nitrite [Aspirols]; metabolized to NO** in vascular smooth muscle.) NO is a **guanylate cyclase activator** that raises the level of cGMP in vascular smooth muscle. Guanylate cyclase catalyzes the conversion of GTP → cGMP, which inhibits Ca^{2+} binding and dephosphorylates the myosin light chain. This leads to vascular smooth muscle relaxation. These drugs are predominantly **venous vasodilators**. This results in: **decreased preload, decreased afterload, and decreased cardiac output, which decreases myocardial O_2 demand**, and **increased myocardial O_2 supply** due to a redistribution of blood flow.

B. Calcium channel antagonists

1. **Nifedipine (Procardia) and Nicardipine (Cardene) are L-type Ca^{2+} channel antagonists** that bind to Ca^{2+} channels and block Ca^+ influx predominantly in vascular smooth muscle. These drugs are **arterial vasodilators**, which increase

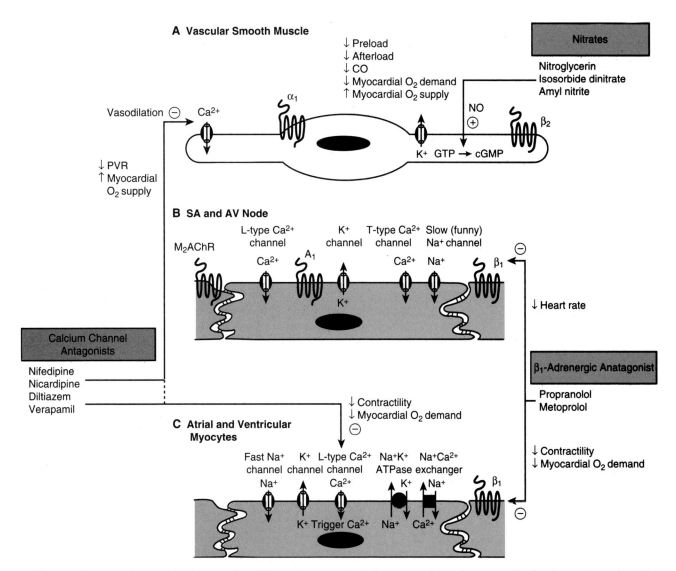

FIGURE 8-3. Diagram of antianginal drug action. (A) Vascular smooth muscle. α_1—α_1 adrenergic receptor; β_2—β_2 adrenergic receptor; CO—cardiac output; PVR—peripheral vascular resistance. **(B)** SA and AV node (slow-response action potential). A_1—A_1 adenosine receptor; M_2AChR—M_2 muscarinic acetylcholine receptor. **(C)** Atrial and ventricular myocytes (fast-response action potential). Note that antianginal drugs are basically used to decrease myocardial O_2 demand or increase myocardial O_2 supply.

myocardial O_2 supply. This results in the following antianginal effect: **decreased PVR. Clinical uses** include: angina, hypertension, and Raynaud's phenomenon.

2. **Diltiazem (Cardizem) and verapamil (Calan, Isoptin, Verelan)** are **L-type Ca^{2+} channel antagonists** that bind to Ca^+ ion channels and block Ca^{2+} influx predominantly in cardiac muscle. These drugs have only mild vasodilatory effects. This results in the following antianginal effects: **decreased contractility of atrial and ventricular myocytes (or negative inotropism)**, which decreases myocardial O_2 demand, and **mildly increased vasodilation**, which increases myocardial O_2 supply. **Clinical uses** include: angina, hypertension, and supraventricular arrhythmias.

C. **β-Adrenergic antagonists**
   1. **Propranolol (Inderal) is a nonselective β_1 and β_2-adrenergic receptor antagonist** that blocks the effects of the sympathetic nervous system on the heart. Remember that postganglionic sympathetic axons innervating the heart release NE. NE binds to the β_1-adrenergic receptor, which is a **G_S-protein–linked receptor** that stimulates the adenylate cyclase and increases cAMP levels. A β-adrenergic receptor antagonist decreases cAMP levels. This results in the following antianginal effects: **decreased contractility of atrial and ventricular myocytes (or negative inotropism)**, which decreases myocardial O_2 demand, and **decreased heart rate (or negative chronotropism)**. **Clinical uses** include: angina, hypertension, supraventricular arrhythmias, ventricular tachycardia, and digitalis-induced arrhythmia.
   2. **Metoprolol (Lopressor)** is a cardioselective **β_1-adrenergic receptor antagonist** and has effects similar to those of propranolol.

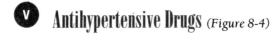

Ⅴ Antihypertensive Drugs *(Figure 8-4)*

A. **α_1-Adrenergic antagonists. Doxazosin (Cardura), prazosin (Minipress), and terazosin (Hytrin)** are **α_1-adrenergic receptor antagonists** that block the effects of the sympathetic nervous system on **arterioles** and **veins**. Remember that postganglionic sympathetic neurons innervating the smooth muscle of blood vessels release NE. NE binds to the α_1-adrenergic receptor, which is a **G_q-protein–liked receptor** that stimulates phospholipase C and increases inositol triphosphate (IP_3) and diacylglycerol (DAG). A α_1-adrenergic receptor antagonist decreases IP_3 and DAG, leading to vasodilation. This results in: **decreased PVR, decreased venous return to the heart, decreased preload,** and **decreased afterload. Clinical uses** include: hypertension and benign prostatic hyperplasia.

B. **Direct vasodilators**
   1. **Hydralazine (Apresoline)** is an **arteriolar vasodilator** that acts directly on vascular smooth muscle (mechanism unknown). This results in: **decreased PVR. Clinical uses** include: CHF and hypertension.
   2. **Minoxidil (Loniten;** a prodrug metabolized to minoxidil sulfate) is a **K^+ channel agonist** that activates K^+ channels and raises K^+ efflux. Minoxidil is an **arteriolar vasodilator** that acts directly on vascular smooth muscle. This results in: **decreased PVR** due to hyperpolarization and relaxation of arteriolar smooth muscle. **Clinical uses** include: CHF and hypertension.

▶

FIGURE 8-4. Diagram of antihypertensive drug action. (A) Vascular smooth muscle. PVR—peripheral vascular resistance. **(B)** Central nervous system (*CNS*). CO—cardiac output. **(C)** Peripheral nervous system (*PNS*). **(D)** Atrial and ventricular myocytes (fast-response action potential). **(E)** Lung capillaries. The endothelium of lung capillaries comprises the major site of angiotensin I → angiotensin II conversion. ACE—angiotensin-converting enzyme. **(F)** Kidney. ATL—ascending thin limb of the loop of Henle; BC—Bowman's capsule; CD—collecting ducts; DCT—distal convoluted tubule; DST—distal straight tubule; DTL—descending thin limb of the loop of Henle; PCT—proximal convoluted tubule.

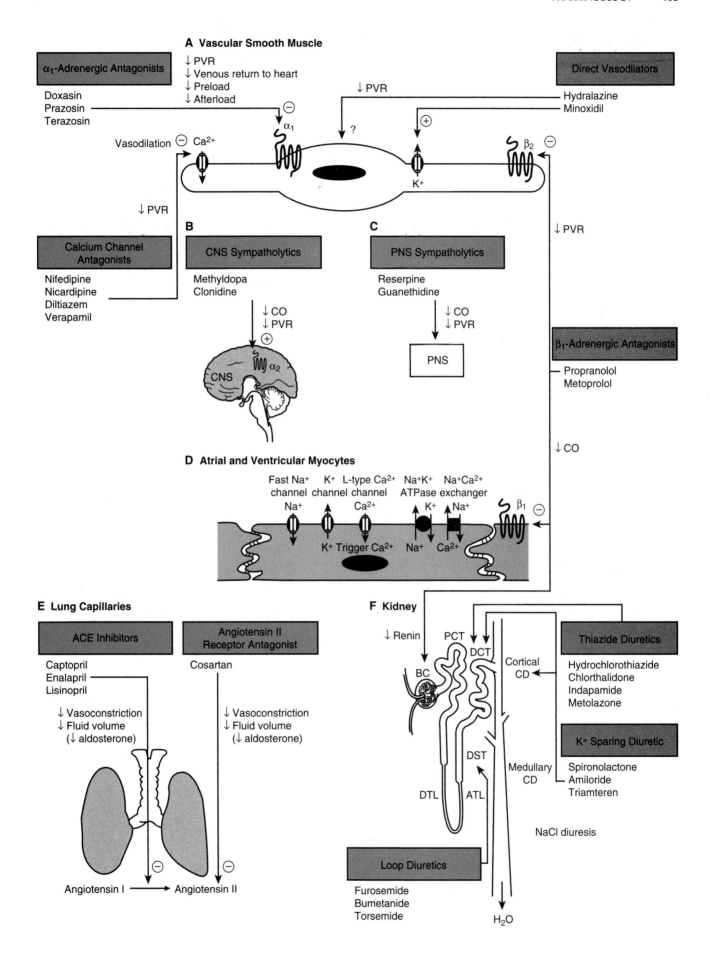

A Vascular Smooth Muscle

α₁-Adrenergic Antagonists

Doxasin
Prazosin
Terazosin

↓ PVR
↓ Venous return to heart
↓ Preload
↓ Afterload

Direct Vasodilators

Hydralazine
Minoxidil

↓ PVR

⊖ α₁

Vasodilation ⊖ Ca²⁺

?

⊕

β₂ ⊖

K⁺

↓ PVR

↓ PVR

Calcium Channel Antagonists

Nifedipine
Nicardipine
Diltiazem
Verapamil

B

CNS Sympatholytics

Methyldopa
Clonidine

↓ CO
↓ PVR
⊕ α₂

CNS

C

PNS Sympatholytics

Reserpine
Guanethidine

↓ CO
↓ PVR

PNS

β₁-Adrenergic Antagonists

Propranolol
Metoprolol

↓ CO

D Atrial and Ventricular Myocytes

Fast Na⁺ channel   K⁺ channel   L-type Ca²⁺ channel   Na⁺K⁺ ATPase   Na⁺Ca²⁺ exchanger

Na⁺   Ca²⁺   K⁺   Na⁺

K⁺ Trigger Ca²⁺   Na⁺   Ca²⁺

β₁ ⊖

E Lung Capillaries

ACE Inhibitors

Captopril
Enalapril
Lisinopril

↓ Vasoconstriction
↓ Fluid volume
(↓ aldosterone)

Angiotensin II Receptor Antagonist

Cosartan

↓ Vasoconstriction
↓ Fluid volume
(↓ aldosterone)

Angiotensin I ⟶ Angiotensin II

⊖   ⊖

F Kidney

↓ Renin

PCT

DCT

BC

Cortical CD

DST

Medullary CD

DTL   ATL

NaCl diuresis

Thiazide Diuretics

Hydrochlorothiazide
Chlorthalidone
Indapamide
Metolazone

K⁺ Sparing Diuretic

Spironolactone
Amiloride
Triamteren

Loop Diuretics

Furosemide
Bumetanide
Torsemide

H₂O

C. Calcium channel antagonists
1. **Nifedipine (Procardia) and nicardipine (Cardene) are L-type Ca^{2+} channel antagonists** that bind to Ca^{2+} channels and block Ca^{2+} influx predominantly in smooth muscle. These drugs are **arterial vasodilators.** This results in the following antihypertensive effect: **decreased PVR. Clinical uses** include: angina, hypertension, and Raynaud's phenomenon.
2. **Diltiazem (Cardizem) and verapamil (Calan, Isoptin, Verelan) are L-type Ca^{2+} channel antagonists** that bind to Ca^{2+} channels and block Ca^{2+} influx predominantly in cardiac muscle. These drugs have only mild vasodilatory effects. This results in the following antihypertensive effect: **decreased PVR** due to mildly increased vasodilation. **Clinical uses** include: angina, hypertension, and supraventricular arrhythmias.

D. **Central nervous system (CNS) sympatholytics. Methyldopa (Aldomet;** a prodrug metabolized to methyl-norepinephrine) and **clonidine (Catapres)** are α$_2$-adrenergic **agonists** that inhibit sympathetic nervous system outflow. This results in: **decreased cardiac output** and **decreased PVR. Clinical use** includes: hypertension.

E. Peripheral Nervous System (PNS) Sympatholytics
1. **Reserpine (Serpasil)** irreversibly binds to neurosecretory vesicles in adrenergic neurons and reduces uptake of NE, dopamine, and serotonin in the PNS (some CNS action). This results in: **decreased cardiac output** and **decreased PVR. Clinical uses** include: hypertension and Huntington's disease.
2. **Guanethidine (Ismelin)** slowly displaces NE in neurosecretory vesicles (substitute neurotransmitter) and blocks the release of NE from adrenergic neurons. This results in: **decreased cardiac output** and **decreased PVR. Clinical use** includes: hypertension.

F. β-Adrenergic antagonists
1. **Propranolol (Inderal)** is a **nonselective β$_1$- and β$_2$-adrenergic receptor antagonist** that blocks the effects of the sympathetic nervous system on the heart and blood vessels. Remember that postganglionic sympathetic axons innervating the heart release NE. NE binds to the β$_1$-adrenergic receptor, which is a **G$_s$-protein–linked receptor** that stimulates the adenylate cyclase and increases cAMP levels. A β-adrenergic receptor antagonist decreases cAMP levels. This results in the following antihypertensive effects: **decreased cardiac output; decreased PVR** due to inhibitory action on CNS centers that control sympathetic outflow to vascular smooth muscle; and **inhibition of renin release by kidney. Clinical uses** include: hypertension, angina, supraventricular arrhythmias, ventricular tachycardia, and digitalis-induced arrhythmia.
2. **Metoprolol (Lopressor)** is a cardioselective **β$_1$-adrenergic receptor antagonist** and has effects similar to those of propranolol.

G. **ACE inhibitors. Captopril (Capoten), enalapril (Vasotec),** and **lisinopril (Prinivil)** are **ACE inhibitors** that reversibly inhibit ACE and prevent the conversion of angiotensin I → angiotensin II (a potent vasoconstrictor), leading to low levels of angiotensin II. This results in: **decreased vasoconstriction** due to the low levels of angiotensin II and **decreased fluid volume** due to low levels of aldosterone (caused by low levels of angiotensin II). **Clinical uses** include: CHF and hypertension.

H. Angiotensin II receptor antagonist. **Losartan (Cozaar;** metabolized to more potent 5-carboxylic acid form) is an **angiotensin II receptor antagonist** that blocks the action of angiotensin II (a potent vasoconstrictor). This results in: **decreased vasoconstriction** due to the blocked action of angiotensin II and **decreased fluid volume** due to low levels of aldosterone (caused by the blocked action of angiotensin II). **Clinical use** includes: hypertension.

I. **Diuretics**

1. **Loop diuretics (sulfonamide derivatives). Furosemide (Lasix), bumetanide (Bumex), and torsemide (Demadex)** are Na^+-K^+-$2Cl^+$ **symporter inhibitors** that act on the **distal straight tubule (DST) of the loop of Henle** and cause a decreased NaCl reabsorption (tubular fluid → plasma). This results in: **NaCl diuresis; hypokalemic alkalosis** due to the delivery of large amounts of Na^+ to the cortical collecting duct causing K^+ secretion (plasma → tubular fluid; K^+ wasting); and H^+ secretion (plasma → tubular fluid). **Clinical uses** include: edema associated with CHF, liver disease, renal disease, and pulmonary disease; hypertension (due to decrease in blood volume).

2. **Thiazide diuretics (sulfonamide derivatives). Hydrochlorothiazide (Hydro-DIURIL), chlorthalidone (Hygroton), indapamide (Lozol), and metolazone (Mykrox)** are Na^+-Cl^- **symporter inhibitors** that act on the early distal convoluted tubule **(DCT)** and cause a decreased NaCl reabsorption (tubular fluid → plasma). This results in: **NaCl diuresis; hypokalemic alkalosis** due to the delivery of large amounts of Na^+ to the cortical collecting duct, causing K^+ secretion (plasma → tubular fluid; K^+ wasting); and H^+ secretion (plasma → tubular fluid). **Clinical uses** include: edema associated with CHF, liver disease, renal disease, and corticosteroid therapy; and hypertension (due to decrease in blood volume).

3. **K^+-sparing diuretics**

    a. **Spironolactone (Aldactone)** is an **aldosterone antagonist** that acts by reducing gene expression of Na^+ channels and Na^+-K^+ ATPase in the cortical collecting ducts. This causes a decreased NaCl reabsorption (tubular fluid → plasma), decreased K^+ secretion (plasma → tubular fluid; K^+ **sparing**), and decreased H^+ secretion (plasma → tubular fluid). This results in: **NaCl diuresis with K^+-sparing. Clinical uses** include: hypertension, edematous states, and primary hyperaldosteronism (Conn's syndrome).

    b. **Amiloride (Midamor) and triamterene (Dyrenium)** are Na^+ **channel antagonists** that block Na^+ channels in the late DCT and collecting ducts. This causes a decreased NaCl reabsorption (tubular fluid → plasma), decreased K^+ secretion (plasma → tubular fluid; K^+ **sparing**), and decreased H^+ secretion (plasma → tubular fluid). This results in: **NaCl diuresis with K^+-sparing. Clinical uses** include: hypertension and edematous states.

J. **Hypertensive emergencies**

1. **Diazoxide (Hyperstat)** is an ATP-sensitive K^+ **ATP channel agonist** that activates K^+ channels and raises K^+ efflux. This causes hyperpolarization of arteriolar smooth muscle cells and results in: **arteriolar vasodilation. Clinical uses** include: hypertensive emergencies.

2. **Sodium nitroprusside (Nitropress;** metabolized to **NO** in vascular smooth muscle). NO is a **guanylate cyclase activator** that raises the level of cGMP in vascular smooth muscle. Guanylate cyclase catalyzes the conversion of GTP → cGMP, which inhibits Ca^+ binding and dephosphorylates the myosin light chain. This leads to vascular smooth muscle relaxation. Sodium nitroprusside is an **arteriolar and venous vasodilator.** This results in: **decreased PVR** due to relaxation of arteriolar and venous smooth muscle; **decreased preload** (load on the ventricular myocytes at the end of diastole); and **decreased afterload** (load on the ventricular myocytes during systole). **Clinical uses** include: CHF and hypertensive emergencies.

3. **Trimethaphan (Arfonad)** is a **nicotinic acetylcholine receptor (nAChR) antagonist** that blocks at the autonomic ganglion where preganglionic axons synapse with postganglionic cell bodies. This causes both a sympathetic block and a parasympathetic block and results in **decreased arterial blood pressure.**

4. **Labetalol (Normodyne)** is an **adrenergic receptor antagonist** that has both α_1-adrenergic blocking action and nonselective β-adrenergic blocking action.

VI **Antithrombotic Drugs** (Table 8-1)

A. Antiplatelet drugs
1. **Aspirin (acetylsalicylic acid; Bayer, Bufferin)** irreversibly inhibits **cyclooxygenase** and causes a decreased production of **thromboxane (TXA_2; a potent stimulator of platelet aggregation).** **Clinical uses** include: antiplatelet, myocardial infarction, analgesia, antipyretic, and anti-inflammatory.
2. **Ticlopidine (Ticlid)** irreversibly inhibits the binding of **fibrinogen to glycoprotein IIb/IIIa complex** located on the platelet membrane. **Clinical use** includes: stroke.
3. **Dipyridamole (Dipridacot)** inhibits platelet aggregation. The mechanism is not fully understood. **Clinical use** includes: thromboemboli.
4. **Sulfinpyrazone (Anturan)** inhibits platelet adherence to subendothelial connective tissue and inhibits platelet secretion. The mechanism is not fully understood. **Clinical uses** include: chronic gout, hyperuricemia, and recurrent myocardial infarction.

B. Anticoagulants
1. **Heparin** increases the proteolytic action of antithrombin III, which inactivates various clotting factors (e.g., factors IIa, IX, X, XI, and XII). **Clinical uses** include: anticoagulant, deep vein thrombosis, pulmonary thromboembolism, and stroke.
2. **Warfarin (Coumadin)** inhibits the synthesis of **vitamin K,** which prevents the carboxylation of glutamic acid residues of clotting factors (e.g., factors II, VII, IX, and X). **Clinical uses** include: deep vein thrombosis and pulmonary thromboembolism.

C. Thrombolytics
1. **Streptokinase (Streptase, Kabikinase)** combines with plasminogen to form an activator complex, which converts plasminogen (free and fibrin-bound) → plasmin.
2. **Eminase (Anistreplase;** anisoylated streptokinase prodrug) is similar to streptokinase.
3. **Tissue plasminogen activator (tPA, Alteplase)** directly converts plasminogen (fibrin-bound only) → plasmin.
4. **Urokinase (Abbokinase)** directly converts plasminogen (free and fibrin-bound) → plasmin.

VII **Antihyperlipidemic Drugs** (Table 8-1)

A. 3-Hydroxy-3-methylglutaryl-coenzyme A (HMG-CoA) reductase inhibitors (lovastatin [Mevacor], simvastatin [Zocor], pravastatin [Pravachol], fluvastatin [Lescol]) reversibly and competitively inhibit **HMG-CoA reductase,** which catalyzes the rate-limiting step in cholesterol synthesis (HMG-CoA → mevalonate). This results in: **increased low-density lipoprotein (LDL) receptors in the liver** and **increased catabolism of LDL.** **Clinical uses** include: type IIa and type IIb hyperlipidemia.

B. Resins (cholestyramine [Questran], colestipol [Colestid]) promote the excretion of bile salts by forming an insoluble complex in the small intestine. This results in: **increased conversion of cholesterol → bile; increased LDL receptors in the liver;** and **increased catabolism of LDL.** **Clinical uses** include: type IIa and type IIb hyperlipidemia.

C. Vitamin B (niacin [nicotinic acid, vitamin B_3]) decreases production of very-low-density lipoproteins (VLDL), leading to decreased LDL levels and increased high-density lipoprotein (HDL) levels by an unknown mechanism. **Clinical uses** include: types IIb, III, IV, and V hyperlipidemia; niacin deficiency; and pellagra.

TABLE 8-1	**SUMMARY TABLE OF DRUGS**
Drug Class	**Drug**
Antiarrhythmic drugs	**Class IA:** Quinidine (Quinaglute, Quinidex), procainamide (Procan-SR, Pronestyl), disopyramide (Norpace) **Class IB:** Lidocaine (Xylocaine), tocainide (Tonocard), mexiletine (Mexitil), phenytoin (Dilantin) **Class 1C:** Flecainide (Tambocor), propafenone (Rythmol), moricizine (Ethmozine) **Class II:** Propranolol (Inderal), metoprolol (Lopressor), esmolol (Brevibloc), sotalol (Betapace) **Class III:** Amiodarone (Cordarone), bretylium (Bretylol) **Class IV:** Diltiazem (Cardizem), verapamil (Calan, Isoptin, Verelan), adenosine (Adenocard)
Congestive heart failure drugs	**Direct vasodilators:** Hydralazine (Apresoline), minoxidil (Loniten), sodium nitroprusside (Nitropress) **PDE inhibitors:** Amrinone (Inocor) and milrinone (Primacor) **Cardiac glycosides:** Digoxin (Lanoxin), digitoxin (Crystodigin) **β-Adrenergic agonist:** Dobutamine (Dobutrex) **ACE inhibitors:** Captopril (Capoten), enalapril (Vasotec), and lisinopril (Prinivil) **Angiotensin II receptor antagonist:** Losartan (Cozaar) **Loop diuretics:** Furosemide (Lasix), bumetanide (Bumex), and torsemide (Demadex) **Thiazide diuretics:** Hydrochlorothiazide (HydroDIURIL), chlorthalidone (Hygroton), indapamide (Lozol), and metolazone (Mykrox)
Antianginal drugs	**Nitrates:** Nitroglycerin (Nitrostat), isosorbide dinitrate (Isordil), amyl nitrite (Aspirols) **Calcium channel antagonists:** Nifedipine (Procardia), nicardipine (Cardene), diltiazem (Cardizem), verapamil (Calan, Isoptin, Verelan) **β-Adrenergic antagonists:** Propranolol (Inderal), metoprolol (Lopressor)
Antihypertensive drugs	**α_1-Adrenergic antagonists:** Doxazosin (Cardura), prazosin (Minipress), terazosin (Hytrin) **Direct vasodilators:** Hydralazine (Apresoline), minoxidil (Loniten) **Calcium channel antagonists:** Nifedipine (Procardia), nicardipine (Cardene), diltiazem (Cardizem), verapamil (Calan, Isoptin, Verelan) **Central nervous system sympatholytics:** Methyldopa (Aldomet) and clonidine (Catapres) **Peripheral nervous system sympatholytics:** Reserpine (Serpasil) and guanethidine (Ismelin) **β-Adrenergic antagonists:** Propranolol (Inderal) and metoprolol (Lopressor) **ACE inhibitors:** Captopril (Capoten), enalapril (Vasotec), and lisinopril (Prinivil) **Angiotensin II receptor antagonist:** Losartan (Cozaar) **Loop diuretics:** Furosemide (Lasix), bumetanide (Bumex), and torsemide (Demadex) **Thiazides diuretics:** Hydrochlorothiazide (HydroDIURIL), chlorthalidone (Hygroton), indapamide (Lozol), and metolazone (Mykrox) **K^+-sparing diuretics:** Spironolactone (Aldactone), amiloride (Midamor), triamterene (Dyrenium)
Hypertensive emergencies	Diazoxide (Hyperstat), sodium nitroprusside (Nitropress), trimethaphan (Arfonad), labetalol (Normodyne)
Antithrombotic drugs	**Antiplatelet drugs:** Aspirin (acetylsalicylic acid; Bayer, Bufferin), ticlopidine (Ticlid), dipyridamole (Dipridacot), sulfinpyrazone (Anturan) **Anticoagulants:** Heparin, warfarin (Coumadin) **Thrombolytics:** Streptokinase (Streptase, Kabikinase), eminase (Anistreplase), tissue plasminogen activator (tPA, Alteplase), urokinase (Abbokinase)
Antihyperlipidemic drugs	**HMG-CoA reductase inhibitors:** Lovastatin (Mevacor), simvastatin (Zocor), pravastatin (Pravachol), fluvastatin (Lescol) **Resins:** Cholestyramine (Questran), colestipol (Colestid) **Vitamin B:** Niacin (nicotinic acid, vitamin B_3)

ACE—angiotensin-converting enzyme; PDE—phosphodiesterase.

Credits

Figure 1-1: A–D Modified from Dudek RW. *BRS Embryology*. 2nd Ed. Baltimore: Lippincott, Williams & Wilkins, 1998:42, 43. **F, G** Modified from Johnson KE, *Human Developmental Anatomy*. Philadelphia: Lippincott Williams & Wilkins, 1988:147.

Figure 1-2: A Redrawn from Dudek RW. *BRS Embryology*. 2nd Ed. Baltimore: Lippincott Williams & Wilkins, 1998:46. **B** Modified from *BRS Embryology*. 2nd Ed. Philadelphia: Lippincott Williams & Wilkins, 1998:49.

Figure 1-3: A Modified from Dudek RW. *High Yield Embryology*. 2nd Ed. Philadelphia: Lippincott Williams & Wilkins, 2001:30. Note change to original picture. **B** Redrawn from Dudek RW. *BRS Embryology*. 2nd Ed. Philadelphia: Lippincott Williams & Wilkins, 1998:50.

Figure 1-4: A Modified from Dudek RW. *BRS Embryology*. 2nd Ed. Philadelphia: Lippincott Williams & Wilkins, 1998:47. **B (a–d)** Modified from Dudek RW. *BRS Embryology*. 2nd Ed. Philadelphia: Lippincott Williams & Wilkins, 1998:52. **B (e)** Redrawn from Dudek RW. *BRS Embryology*. 2nd Ed. Philadelphia: Lippincott Williams & Wilkins, 1998:52.

Figure 1-5: A Modified from Dudek RW. *BRS Embryology*. 2nd Ed. Philadelphia: Lippincott Williams & Wilkins, 1998:47. **B** Redrawn from Allen HD, Gutgesell HP, Clark EB, Driscoll DJ, eds. *Moss and Adams' Heart Disease in Infants, Children, and Adolescents,* vol. 1, 6th Ed. Philadelphia: Lippincott Williams & Wilkins, 2001:637.

Figure 1-6: A, B Redrawn from Johnson KE. *Human Developmental Anatomy*. Baltimore: Williams & Wilkins, 1988:154.

Figure 1-7: A–C Redrawn from Johnson KE. *Human Developmental Anatomy*. Baltimore: Williams & Wilkins, 1988:158.

Figure 1-8: A-D Modified from Lucas RV, Anderson RC, Amplatz K, et al. Congenital causes of pulmonary venous obstruction. Pediatr Clin North Am 1963: 781–836. **E (a, b)** Modified from Edwards JE. Symposium on anomalous pulmonary venous connection: pathologic and developmental considerations in anomalous pulmonary venous connection. Proc Staff Meetings Mayo Clin 1953;28: 441–452.

Figure 1-9: Adapted from Dudek RW. *High Yield Embryology*. 2nd Ed. Philadelphia: Lippincott Williams & Wilkins, 2001:24.

Figure 1-10: A, B From Kirks DR. *Practical Pediatric Imaging*. 3rd Ed. Baltimore: Williams & Wilkins, 1997:630. **C** From Kirks DR. *Practical Pediatric Imaging*. 3rd Ed. Baltimore: Williams & Wilkins, 1997:631.

Figure 1-11: A, B From Swischuk LE. *Imaging of the Newborn, Infant, and Young Child*. 5th Ed. Philadelphia: Lippincott Williams & Wilkins, 2004:258, 261. **C** From Valdes-Cruz LM, Cayre RO. *Echocardiographic Diagnosis of Congenital Heart Disease*. Philadelphia: Lippincott Williams & Wilkins, 1999:451. **D** From Kirks DR. *Practical Pediatric Imaging*. 3rd Ed. Baltimore: Williams & Wilkins, 1997:557. **E** From Swischuk LE. *Imaging of the Newborn, Infant, and Young Child*. 5th Ed. Philadelphia: Lippincott Williams & Wilkins, 2004:264. **F** From Kirks DR. *Practical Pediatric Imaging*. 3rd Ed. Baltimore: Williams & Wilkins, 1997:558. **G** From Allen HD, Gutgesell HP, Clark EB, Driscoll DJ, eds. *Moss and Adams' Heart Disease in Infants, Children, and Adolescents*, vol. 1, 6th Ed. Philadelphia: Lippincott Williams & Wilkins, 2001:1107. Courtesy of Williams D. Edwards. **H** From Valdes-Cruz LM, Cayre RO. *Echocardiographic Diagnosis of Congenital Heart Disease*. Philadelphia: Lippincott Williams & Wilkins, 1999:415. **I** Reprinted with permission from Sridaromont S, Ritter D, Feldt RH, et al. Double-outlet right ventricle: anatomic and angiocardiographic correlations. Mayo Clin Proc

1978; 53:555–577. **J** From Kirks DR. *Practical Pediatric Imaging*. 3rd Ed. Baltimore: Williams & Wilkins, 1997:547. **K, L** From Swischuk LE. *Imaging of the Newborn, Infant, and Young Child*. 5th Ed. Philadelphia: Lippincott Williams & Wilkins, 2004:272, 271. **M** From Allen HD, Gutgesell HP, Clark EB, Driscoll DJ, eds. *Moss and Adams' Heart Disease in Infants, Children, and Adolescents*, vol. 1, 6th Ed. Philadelphia: Lippincott Williams & Wilkins, 2001:975. **N** From Allen HD, Gutgesell HP, Clark EB, Driscoll DJ, eds. *Moss and Adams' Heart Disease in Infants, Children, and Adolescents*, vol. 1, 6th Ed. Philadelphia: Lippincott Williams & Wilkins, 2001:977. **O** From Valdes-Cruz LM, Cayre RO. *Echocardiographic Diagnosis of Congenital Heart Disease*. Philadelphia: Lippincott Williams & Wilkins, 1999:383.

Figure 1-12: A From Swischuk LE. *Imaging of the Newborn, Infant, and Young Child*. 5th Ed. Philadelphia: Lippincott Williams & Wilkins, 2004:243. **B** From Pohost GM, O'Rourke RA, Berman DS, Shah PM. *Imaging in Cardiovascular Disease*. Philadelphia: Lippincott Williams & Wilkins, 2000:772. **C** From Swischuk LE. *Imaging of the Newborn, Infant, and Young Child*. 5th Ed. Philadelphia: Lippincott Williams & Wilkins, 2004:244. **D** From Valdes-Cruz LM, Cayre RO. *Echocardiographic Diagnosis of Congenital Heart Disease*. Philadelphia: Lippincott Williams & Wilkins, 1999:192.

Figure 1-13: A, B From Swischuk LE. *Imaging of the Newborn, Infant, and Young Child*. 5th Ed. Philadelphia: Lippincott Williams & Wilkins, 2004:244, 245. **C** From Valdes-Cruz LM, Cayre RO. *Echocardiographic Diagnosis of Congenital Heart Disease*. Philadelphia: Lippincott Williams & Wilkins, 1999:217. **D** From Kirks DR. *Practical Pediatric Imaging*, 3rd Ed. Baltimore: Williams & Wilkins, 1997:555. **E, F** From Swischuk LE. *Imaging of the Newborn, Infant, and Young Child*. 5th Ed. Philadelphia: Lippincott Williams & Wilkins, 2004:277, 278. **G–J** From Allen HD, Gutgesell HP, Clark EB, Driscoll DJ, eds. *Moss and Adams' Heart Disease in Infants, Children, and Adolescents*, vol. 1, 6th Ed. Philadelphia: Lippincott Williams & Wilkins, 2001:1137, 1139. **K, L** From Kirks DR. *Practical Pediatric Imaging*. 3rd Ed. Baltimore: Williams & Wilkins, 1997:553.

Figure 1-14: A From Kirks DR. *Practical Pediatric Imaging*. 3rd Ed. Baltimore: Williams & Wilkins, 1997:519. **B** Courtesy of RM Peshock, MD. **C** From Swischuk LE. *Imaging of the Newborn, Infant, and Young Child*. 5th Ed. Philadelphia: Lippincott Williams & Wilkins, 2004:247. **D** From Valdes-Cruz LM, Cayre RO. *Echocardiographic Diagnosis of Congenital Heart Disease*. Philadelphia: Lippincott Williams & Wilkins, 1999:211.

Figure 1-15: A–C From Swischuk LE. *Imaging of the Newborn, Infant, and Young Child*. 5th Ed. Philadelphia: Lippincott Williams & Wilkins, 2004:297, 298, 299. **D** From Kirks DR. *Practical Pediatric Imaging*. 3rd Ed. Baltimore: Williams & Wilkins, 1997:589.

Figure 1-16: A, B From Swischuk LE. *Imaging of the Newborn, Infant, and Young Child*. 5th Ed. Philadelphia: Lippincott Williams & Wilkins, 2004:305. **C** From Swischuk LE. *Imaging of the Newborn, Infant, and Young Child*. 5th Ed. Philadelphia: Lippincott Williams & Wilkins, 2004:309. **E** From Sunderland CO, Lees MH, Bonchek LI, et al. Congenital pulmonary artery-subclavian steal. J Pediatrics 1972;81:927–931, with permission from Elsevier. **F–H** From Swischuk LE. *Imaging of the Newborn, Infant, and Young Child*. 5th Ed. Philadelphia: Lippincott Williams & Wilkins, 2004: 247, 248, 303. **I** From Kirks DR. *Practical Pediatric Imaging*. 3rd Ed. Baltimore: Williams & Wilkins, 1998:567. **J** From Swischuk LE. *Imaging of the Newborn, Infant, and Young Child*. 5th Ed. Philadelphia: Lippincott Williams & Wilkins, 2004:286. **K** From Kirks DR. *Practical Pediatric Imaging*. 3rd Ed. Baltimore: Williams & Wilkins, 1998:568.

Figure 1-17: A From Swischuk LE. *Imaging of the Newborn, Infant, and Young Child*. 5th Ed. Philadelphia: Lippincott Williams & Wilkins, 2004:319. **B** From Allen HD, Gutgesell HP, Clark EB, Driscoll DJ, eds. *Moss and Adams' Heart Disease in Infants, Children, and Adolescents*, vol. 1, 6th Ed. Philadelphia: Lippincott Williams & Wilkins, 2001:780. **C** From Swischuk LE. *Imaging of the Newborn, Infant, and Young Child*. 5th Ed. Philadelphia: Lippincott Williams & Wilkins, 2004:319.

Figure 1-18: A From Swischuk LE. *Imaging of the Newborn, Infant, and Young Child*. 5th Ed. Philadelphia: Lippincott Williams & Wilkins, 2004:251. **B** From Valdes-Cruz LM, Cayre RO. *Echocardiographic Diagnosis of Congenital Heart Disease*. Philadelphia: Lippincott Williams & Wilkins, 1999:515. **C** From Swischuk LE. *Imaging of the Newborn, Infant, and Young Child*. 5th Ed. Philadelphia: Lippincott Williams & Wilkins, 2004:254. **D** From Allen HD, Gutgesell HP, Clark EB, Driscoll DJ, eds. *Moss and Adams' Heart Disease in Infants, Children, and Adolescents*, vol. 1, 6th Ed. Philadelphia: Lippincott Williams & Wilkins, 2001:746.

Figure 2-1: A Adapted from Moore KL. *Clinically Oriented Anatomy*. 3rd Ed. Baltimore: Williams & Wilkins, 1992:38. **B–D** From Brandt WE, Helms CA. *Fundamentals of Diagnostic Radiology*. 2nd Ed. Philadelphia: Lippincott Williams & Wilkins, 1999:579 582, 596.

Figure 2-2: A Adapted from Moore KL. *Clinically Oriented Anatomy*. 3rd Ed. Baltimore: Williams & Wilkins, 1992:57. **Inset** Adapted from Chen H, Sonneday CJ, Lillemoe KD, eds. *Manual of Common Bedside Surgical Procedures*. 2nd Ed. Philadelphia: Lippincott Williams & Wilkins, 2000:123. **B, C** From Dudek DW. *High Yield Gross Anatomy*. 2nd Ed. Philadelphia: Lippincott Williams & Wilkins, 2002:30. **D** From Daffner RH. *Clinical Radiology: The Essentials*. 2nd Ed. Philadelphia: Lippincott Williams & Wilkins, 1999:93.

Figure 2-3: A From Allen HD, et al., eds. *Moss and Adam's Heart Disease in Infants, Children, and Adolescents*, vol. I, 6th Ed. Philadelphia: Lippincott Williams & Wilkins, 2001:86. **B** Allen HD, et al., eds. *Moss and Adam's Heart Disease in Infants, Children, and Adolescents*, vol. I; 6th Ed. Philadelphia: Lippincott Williams & Wilkins, 2001:86. **C** Adapted from Allen HD, et al., eds. *Moss and Adam's Heart Disease in Infants, Children, and Adolescents*, vol. I, 6th Ed. Philadelphia: Lippincott Williams & Wilkins, 2001:100. **D** Adapted from Allen HD, et al., eds. *Moss and Adam's Heart Disease in Infants, Children, and Adolescents*, vol. I, 6th Ed. Philadelphia: Lippincott Williams & Wilkins, 2001:86.

Figure 2-4: A, B, D, E Adapted from Dudek RW. *High Yield Gross Anatomy*. 2nd Ed. Baltimore: Lippincott Williams & Wilkins, 2002:46.

Figure 2-6: A–H From Allen HD, et al., eds. *Moss and Adam's Heart Disease in Infants, Children, and Adolescents*, vol. I, 6th Ed. Baltimore: Lippincott Williams & Wilkins, 2001:84–85.

Figure 3-1: A–D From Daffner RH. *Clinical Radiology: The Essentials*. 2nd Ed. Philadelphia: Lippincott Williams & Wilkins, 1999:194.

Figure 3-2: A–I From Goodman LR. *Felson's Principles of Chest Roentgenology*. 2nd Ed. Philadelphia: WB Saunders, 1999:202, 204, 206, 208, with permission from Elsevier.

Figure 3-3: A, B Adapted from Pohost GM, et al. *Imaging in Cardiovascular Disease*. Philadelphia: Lippincott Williams & Wilkins, 2000:355. **C, D** Adapted from Pohost GM, et al. *Imaging in Cardiovascular Disease*. Philadelphia: Lippincott Williams & Wilkins, 2000:354.

Figure 3-4: A–C Adapted from Topol EJ, ed. *Textbook of Cardiovascular Medicine*. 2nd Ed. Philadelphia: Lippincott Williams & Wilkins, 2002:1093.

Figure 3-5: A–F Adapted from Barrett CP, et al. *Primer of Sectional Anatomy with MRI and CT Correlation*. 2nd Ed. Philadelphia: Lippincott Williams & Wilkins, 1994:59, 61, 63, 65, 67, 69.

Figure 4-1: B Modified from Ross MH, Kaye GI, Pawlina W. *Histology: A Text and Atlas*. 4th Ed. Philadelphia: Lippincott Williams & Wilkins, 2003:262. **C** From Ross MH, Kaye GI, Pawlina W. *Histology: A Text and Atlas*. 4th Ed. Philadelphia: Lippincott Williams & Wilkins, 2003:277. **D** Courtesy of Don W. Fawcett, MD. **E** From Dieter Dellman H et al. *Veterinary Histology*. 5th Ed. Philadelphia: Lippincott Williams & Wilkins, 1998:89. Courtesy of WS Tyler. **F** From Dudek RW. *High Yield Histology*. 3rd Ed. Baltimore: Lippincott Williams & Wilkins, 2004:100. Courtesy of Dr. RW Dudek.

Figure 4-2: From Eroschenko VP. *DiFiore's Atlas of Histology with Functional Correlations*. 10th Ed. Philadelphia: Lippincott Williams & Wilkins, 2005.

Figure 5-4: A Modified from Constanzo LS. *BRS Physiology*. 3rd Ed. Philadelphia: Lippincott Williams & Wilkins, 2003:97. **B–E** Modified from Bulock J, Boyle J, Wang MB. *NMS Physiology*. 4th Ed. Philadelphia: Lippincott Williams & Wilkins, 2001:161–162.

Figure 5-5: A, B Modified from Dudek RW. *High Yield Histology*. 3rd Ed. Philadelphia: Lippincott Williams & Wilkins, 2004:90.

Figure 5-6: Modified from Dudek RW. *High Yield Histology*. 3rd Ed. Philadelphia: Lippincott Williams & Wilkins, 2004:92.

Figure 6-1: From Dudek RW. *High Yield Histology.* 3rd Ed. Philadelphia: Lippincott Williams & Wilkins, 2004:102.

Figure 6-2: A Modified from Damjanov I. *High Yield Pathology.* Philadelphia: Lippincott Williams & Wilkins, 2001:38. **C** Modified from Dudek RW. *High Yield Histology.* 3rd Ed. Philadelphia: Lippincott Williams & Wilkins, 2004:92. **D** From Damjanov I, McCue PA, Chansky M. *Histopathology: A Color Atlas and Textbook.* Baltimore: Williams & Wilkins, 1996:101.

Figure 6-3: A From Brandt WE, Helms CA. *Fundamentals of Diagnostic Radiology.* 2nd Ed. Philadelphia: Lippincott Williams & Wilkins, 1999:374. **B** Modified from Collins J, Stern EJ. *Chest Radiology: The Essentials.* Philadelphia: Lippincott Williams & Wilkins, 1999:263. **C** From Brandt WE, Helms CA. *Fundamentals of Diagnostic Radiology.* 2nd Ed. Philadelphia: Lippincott Williams & Wilkins, 1999:364. **D** Brandt WE, Helms CA. *Fundamentals of Diagnostic Radiology.* 2nd Ed. Philadelphia: Lippincott Williams & Wilkins, 1999:532.

Figure 6-4: A–C Modified with permission from Damjanov I, McCue PA, Chansky M. *Histopathology: A Color Atlas and Textbook.* Baltimore: Williams & Wilkins, 1996:108. **B1** From Rubin E, Farber JL. *Pathology.* 3rd Ed. Philadelphia: Lippincott Williams & Wilkins, 1999:578. **B2** From Pohost GM, O'Rourke RA, Berman DS, Shah PM. *Imaging in Cardiovascular Disease.* Philadelphia: Lippincott Williams & Wilkins, 2000:659. **B3, B4** From Sternberg SS. *Diagnostic Surgical Pathology,* vol. 1, 3rd Ed. Philadelphia: Lippincott Williams & Wilkins, 1999:1212. **C** Modified with permission from Damjanov I, McCue PA, Chansky M. *Histopathology: A Color Atlas and Textbook.* Baltimore: Williams & Wilkins, 1996:108. **C1** From Rugin E, Farber JL. *Pathology.* 3rd Ed. Philadelphia: Lippincott Williams & Wilkins, 1999. **C2** From Damjanov I, McCue PA, Chansky M. *Histopathology: A Color Atlas and Textbook.* Baltimore: Williams & Wilkins, 1996:109. **D** Modified with permission from Damjanov I, McCue PA, Chansky M. *Histopathology: A Color Atlas and Textbook.* Baltimore: Williams & Wilkins, 1996:108. **D1, D2** From Damjanov I, McCue PA, Chansky M. *Histopathology: A Color Atlas and Textbook.* Baltimore: Williams & Wilkins, 1996:109.

Figure 6-5: A From Rubin E, Farber JL. *Pathology.* 3rd Ed. Philadelphia: Lippincott Williams & Wilkins, 1999:574. **B, C** From Rubin E, Farber JL. *Pathology.* 3rd Ed. Philadelphia: Lippincott Williams & Wilkins, 1999:573. **D** From Virmani R, Burke AP, Farb A. *Atlas of Cardiovascular Pathology.* Philadelphia: WB Saunders, 1996:64–68, with permission from Elsevier. **E** From Alpert JS, Dalen JE, Rahimtooola SH. *Valvular Heart Disease.* 3rd Ed. Philadelphia: Lippincott Williams & Wilkins, 2000:10.

Figure 7-1: A, B Modified from Rubin E, Farber JL. *Pathology.* 3rd Ed. Philadelphia: Lippincott Williams & Wilkins, 1999:569. **C** From Rubin E, Farber JL. *Pathology.* 3rd Ed. Philadelphia: Lippincott Williams & Wilkins, 1999:570.

Figure 7-2: A–C From Alpert JS, Dalen JE, Rahimtooola SH. *Valvular Heart Disease.* 3rd Ed. Philadelphia: Lippincott Williams & Wilkins, 2000:28.

Figure 7-3: B, D From Damjanov I, McCue PA, Chansky M. *Histopathology: A Color Atlas and Textbook.* Baltimore: Williams & Wilkins, 1996:106.

Index